Instructor's Resource Manual to Accompany

Basic Concepts of Psychiatric- Mental Health Nursing

FIFTH EDITION

Louise Rebraca Shives

Prepared by
Carol J. Cornwell, PhD, RN, CS
Assistant Professor of Nursing
Director, Center for Nursing Scholarship
ANA Certified Adult Psychiatric Mental Health
Clinical Nurse Specialist
Georgia Southern University
School of Nursing
Statesboro, Georgia

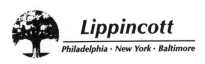
Lippincott
Philadelphia · New York · Baltimore

Ancillary Editor: Doris S. Wray
Senior Production Manager: Helen Ewan
Production Editor: Debra Schiff

Fifth edition

ISBN: 0-7817-2876-2

Any procedure or practice described in this book should be applied by the health care practitioner under appropriate supervision in accordance with professional standards of care used with regard to the unique circumstances that apply in each practice situation. Care has been taken to confirm the accuracy of information presented and to describe generally accepted practices. However, the authors, editors, and publisher cannot accept any responsibility for errors or omissions or for any consequences from application of the information in this book and make no warranty, express or implied, with respect to the contents of the book. Every effort has been made to ensure drug selections and dosages are in accordance with current recommendations and practice. Because of ongoing research, changes in government regulations, and the constant flow of information on drug therapy, reactions, and interactions, the reader is cautioned to check the package insert for each drug for indications, dosages, warnings, and precautions, particularly if the drug is new or infrequently used.

Preface

Teaching psychiatric and mental health nursing is both a challenging and rewarding experience. As health care has become more complex, and connections between the brain, behavior, and healing are increasingly elucidated, it is more important than ever to attend to the mental health needs of clients when delivering nursing care in a multitude of settings. This Fifth Edition of the *Instructor's Resource Manual* has been revised to reflect current trends and recent changes in the mental health care environment. As Internet capabilities have expanded and resources are readily available to professional nurses and nursing students in home, school, and work settings, so too must the breadth and scope of written instructional materials.

This manual has been designed to assist instructors of psychiatric nursing in the education of entry-level nursing students in a wide range of nursing programs and settings. It accompanies *Basic Concepts of Psychiatric–Mental Health Nursing*, Fifth Edition, by Louise Rebraca Shives and has been revised to correspond with the new edition. Each chapter of the *Instructor's Resource Manual* includes the following sections:

- **A Chapter Summary and Outline:** to provide the instructor with an overview of chapter materials and to assist in the development of classroom presentations.

- **Key Words:** that may require definition, discussion, and clarification with students.

- **Teaching Strategies:** pedagogical techniques designed to assist the instructor with the preparation of materials that will enhance student learning and application of chapter concepts and skills to clinical experiences.

- **Test Items:** written in the format consistent with the National Council Licensure Examination for Registered Nurses (NCLEX). Multiple choice questions cover the five steps of the nursing process (Assessment, Analysis, Planning, Implementation, and Evaluation) and the four categories of client needs (Safe, Effective Care Environment; Physiological Integrity; Psychosocial Integrity; and Health Promotion and Maintenance). The testbank was designed to be a supplemental aid for faculty; additional items may be added to provide detail that may be specific to a nursing program or student population.

• Images from textbook

   There are two appendices in the *Instructor's Resource Manual.* Appendix A contains a list of media sources and selected Internet sites that may be beneficial to faculty as they prepare the course. Appendix B contains an example of an Interpersonal Process Analysis (IPA) that may be useful in the clinical setting, or as an aid in the classroom for illustrating clinical scenarios. Both blank and completed IPAs are included in Appendix B.

■ Classroom and Clinical Education in Psychiatric–Mental Health Nursing

OBJECTIVES AND OUTCOMES

In preparing for classroom presentation and clinical experiences, creativity and flexibility are a must. Students are adult learners, who come to the classroom and clinical settings with a wide variety of learning styles. Effective learning experiences are those that provide a mix of activities that allow learners to use their specific learning style and strategies in the application of psychiatric mental health concepts. Preparing objectives and desired outcomes for each classroom and clinical experience is a must for the organized instructor. Objectives with associated student outcomes provide a blueprint for presenting and incorporating materials into classrooms and clinical experiences. In addition, they allow the student to focus on the main points and significant concepts, and provide an outline for study when preparing for examinations.

STRATEGIES FOR TEACHING

Didactic lectures are increasingly becoming a thing of the past as we move into the technology era and have more interesting and interactive methodologies available for use in the classroom. Often Power-Point slides and other visual methods are useful. The blackboard is always a standard visual tool that can help draw attention to important concepts. Role-playing, games, debates, and student presentations can also help to engage the learner in his/her own learning process during the classroom time. It is not unusual to also have web-supported structures to augment classroom activities. The range and scope of strategies that can be useful for teaching content is limited only by the creativity and imagination of the instructor. This *Instructor's Resource Manual* will provide a variety of teaching methodologies and strategies that may be useful in getting basic concepts of psychiatric mental health nursing across to the adult learner.

Films, videotapes, and case studies are important components that can lend a fresh approach to illustrating psychiatric illnesses and behaviors. Some resources for appropriate media, as well as selected websites, are listed in Appendix A.

LEARNING STYLES

Adult learners bring a wealth of life experience and philosophies to the classroom. Learning styles include, but are not limited to, aural (hearing), print (reading), interactive (speaking), visual (seeing), haptic (hands-on), kinesthetic (physical activity), and olfactory (smelling).[1,2] It is challenging to prepare classroom and clinical activities that will engage students with a variety of learning styles into the active process of discussing and incorporating psychiatric and mental health concepts. A variety of techniques will be presented in this manual to assist instructors in this task.

APPLICATION TO CLINICAL

A unique element of nursing education is the concept of application to clinical experiences. Nursing is a clinical practice, and, therefore, educative strategies in nursing must be aimed toward assisting students to take concepts from the classroom and apply them to clinical scenarios. Oftentimes, this transfer presents a challenge for nursing instruction. Particularly when classroom instruction time is limited, the transfer of theoretical concepts to clinical activities can be challenging, and requires creativity and flexibility on the part of the faculty member. Strategies for doing this are included in each chapter of the *Instructor's Resource Manual*.

INTERPERSONAL PROCESS ANALYSIS TOOL

Psychiatric–mental health nursing education includes the important component of assisting the student to examine his/her own style of interpersonal relationships, communication, thoughts, feelings, and interactions. Traditionally, the Interpersonal Process Analysis (IPA) has been used in psychiatric–mental health nursing as a way to assist the student in developing the skill of self-reflection. The student writes verbatim notes immediately after an interaction has taken place. The student records his/her verbal and nonverbal communication, the client's verbal and nonverbal communication, and identifies whether the responses are therapeutic or not, keeping in mind both the emotions and milieu.

Appendix B contains a blank IPA form that may be used in the clinical setting. In addition, an IPA that has been thoroughly completed is provided as a model for students. The IPA is typically assigned with the following directions for the student:

1. Each IPA must record a minimum of 15-minutes' interaction, not counting introductions.
2. Make sure that for each IPA you submit, you also write brief before and after paragraphs. In these paragraphs, describe:
   (a) the setting in which the interaction was taking place (eg, where were you and the patient?; what were you doing?; and was anything going on that may have affected your interaction?).
   (b) how the interaction ended.

The instructor may feel free to utilize these forms in whatever way would best assist him or her in teaching students the art of self-reflection.

Carol Cornwell

REFERENCES

1. http://www.howtolearn.com/personal.html
2. http://www.learningstyles.org/SevenStylesOverview.htm

Contents

UNIT 5
Clients With Psychiatric Disorders

UNIT 6
Special Populations

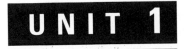
UNIT 1

Psychiatric-Mental Health Nursing

CHAPTER 1

Mental Health and Mental Illness

■ Chapter Summary

This chapter is an overview of concepts about the use of the self in psychiatric–mental health nursing, definitions, misconceptions, factors influencing mental health and mental illness, and strategies for attaining and maintaining mental health. Self-awareness is discussed as a key element to understanding oneself, to examining one's own beliefs and behaviors, and in working with clients who have a variety of clinical symptoms. Mental health and mental illness are defined and discussed. Mental health is a positive state in which the individual is able to be responsible and self-aware, to problem-solve and cope with daily life, and to be generally satisfied with one's life. Mental illness can be caused by interactions between chemical imbalances in the brain, organic brain changes, inherited characteristics, childhood experiences, and life circumstances. Characteristics of mental health are defined, using Maslow's "hierarchy of human needs," which, when met, potentiate the individual's self-actualization and mental health. Powell's five levels of interpersonal communication are presented. Ego defense mechanisms, significant others, and individual personal coping strategies are described as elements that help individuals to attain and maintain mental health.

■ Chapter Outline

I. SELF-AWARENESS
   A. Self-awareness is an effective tool in working with clients who are anxious, depressed, psychotic, or confused.
   B. Individuals have unique personality traits they bring to their interpersonal relationships.
   C. Introspection is the ability to look at oneself, and examine one's own attitudes, beliefs, and behaviors.
   D. Self-awareness results from introspection, and expands the nurse's ability to understand the feelings and behaviors of clients with a variety of clinical symptoms.

II. MENTAL HEALTH

 A. Definition: Mental health is a positive state in which a person is responsible; displays self-awareness; is self-directive; can cope with daily tension and crises and can function well in society; is accepted within a group; is generally satisfied with and enjoys life; fulfills one's capacity for love and work; can become independent, interdependent, or dependent without permanently losing independence; and functions within one's cultural or ethnic group norms.

 B. Factors influencing mental health
   1. Inherited Characteristics: Genetic makeup, or innate differences in sensitivity and temperament, influences mental health and can predispose one to cognitive disability or mental disorders.
   2. Nurturing During Childhood: Familial-child interactions affect mental health, and positive or negative nurturing can profoundly influence the way in which one interacts with others.
   3. Life Circumstances: Positive and negative life circumstances and events significantly influence mental health and can predispose one to mental disorders.

 C. Characteristics of mental health (Maslow, 1970)
   Maslow identified a "hierarchy of needs," including five levels of human need in order to self-actualize: 1) Physiologic (oxygen, food, water, rest, elimination, sex), 2) Security and Safety (shelter, freedom from harm), 3) Love (affection, belongingness, meaningful relations), 4) Self-esteem (being well thought of by self and others), and 5) Self-actualization (self-fulfillment, learning, creativity, reaching one's potential). Mentally healthy individuals are able to accept themselves and others, to form close relationships, to perceive the world and people as they really are, to appreciate and enjoy life, and to be independent and autonomous in thought and action, creative and flexible in problem solving, to demonstrate consistent behavior, respect others, and appreciate differences.

 D. Ways to maintain mental health
   Factors that influence the ability to achieve and maintain mental health include:
   1. Interpersonal Communication:
     Five levels of communication that affect personal growth and maturity during interpersonal encounters (Powell, 1969):
     a. Level 5: Cliché conversation
     b. Level 4: Reporting facts
     c. Level 3: Revealing ideas and judgments
     d. Level 2: Spontaneous here-and-now emotions
     e. Level 1: Open, honest communication
   2. Ego Defense Mechanisms:
     Mental processes first described by Sigmund Freud—usually

unconscious, protective barriers—can be used therapeutically or pathologically to resolve a mental conflict, to reduce anxiety or fear, to protect one's self-esteem, or to protect one's sense of security.

Defense mechanisms are categorized in a variety of ways—sophisticated to primitive, most to least frequently used—and can be healthy or unhealthy, depending on the circumstances in which they are used. Commonly used defense mechanisms are: suppression, repression, rationalization, identification, compensation, reaction-formation, substitution, displacement, restitution or undoing, projection, symbolization, regression, sublimation, denial, introjection, conversion, fantasy, isolation, dissociation, and intellectualization.

3. Significant Others or Support People:
   Significant others or support people can be helpful to buffer against the adverse effects of stress or anxiety. It is important to identify significant others/support people for clients during times of increased distress.
4. Personal Strategies:
   Many individual personal strategies may be useful during stressful times. For example, aerobic exercise, aromatherapy, martial arts, massage, meditation, progressive relaxation, walking, and yoga are unique, personal coping strategies.

III. MENTAL ILLNESS
   A. Definition: Mental illness has been defined as a syndrome or illness with psychological or behavioral manifestations due to social, psychological, genetic, physical/chemical, or biological disturbance, and not limited to relations between the person and society (American Psychiatric Association, 2000). Mental illness can be caused by chemical imbalances, organic changes, or transfer of drugs across placental barrier; and can be influenced by inherited characteristics, childhood experiences, and life circumstances.
   B. Misconceptions about Mental Illness: Several misconceptions have been identified about mental illness (Altrocci, 1980):
      1. Abnormal behavior is different or odd, easily recognized.
      2. Abnormal behavior can be predicted and evaluated.
      3. Internal forces are responsible for abnormal behavior.
      4. People who exhibit abnormal behavior are dangerous.
      5. Maladaptive behavior is always inherited.
      6. Mental illness is incurable.

KEY WORDS

Coping strategies
Ego defense mechanisms
Hierarchy of human needs
Interpersonal communication levels
Introspection
Maladaptive behavior

Mental health
Mental illness
Self-actualization
Self-awareness
Significant others

■ Classroom Teaching Strategies

1. Distribute blank index cards to students. Ask each student to write anonymously a recent life circumstance that created stress for him or her. Gather up the cards, shuffle, and redistribute a card to each student. Have each student give an example of one adaptive and one maladaptive coping mechanism that could be used to deal with the stressor identified on the card he or she received. During the discussion, note trends and similarities in coping mechanisms that students identify, and why they are adaptive versus maladaptive. Identify that some coping mechanisms may be adaptive in some situations and maladaptive in others.

2. Divide the classroom into two groups, instructing Group 1 to use any creative techniques they wish to illustrate the definition of mental health and Group 2 to do the same for mental illness. Encourage students to be creative, using role playing, the blackboard, props, and any other means available. When both groups have presented, compare and contrast the concepts that were illustrated, and discuss the differences between mental health and mental illness.

3. Provide students with a piece of paper that is blank except for a 10-inch line, divided into a Likert scale from 1 to 10; 1 = no self-awareness and 10 = most self-awareness possible. Have students place an "X" along the line where they perceive themselves to be at the current time. Ask students to provide a reason why they selected that number along the line, as well as characteristics they consider to be present when one is "self-aware." Use this exercise to elicit a discussion about the elements of a person's behavior, beliefs, and life circumstances that may contribute to and enhance one's self-awareness.

4. Divide the classroom into five groups, each representing one of Maslow's levels of human need: 1) physiologic, 2) security/safety, 3) love, 4) self-esteem, and 5) self-actualization. Have each group devise a creative portrayal of each level in any way they wish. When they have done so, line up the groups from lowest need to highest, and have each group present their portrayal and discuss why an individual might need to meet lower-level needs in order to progress to higher-level needs.

5. Using 20 index cards, write one ego defense mechanism on each card. Divide students into pairs, distributing one card, face down, to each pair of students. Give students 15 minutes to prepare a brief presentation, with each pair of students illustrating the defense mechanism on the card in front of them, using the board, role-playing, speaking, and any other creative technique. Have the pair demonstrate their defense mechanism to the class, and have the class guess which defense mechanism is being portrayed.

CHAPTER 2

Psychiatric–Mental Health Nursing: History and Trends

■ Chapter Summary

This chapter reviews the specialization of psychiatric–mental health nursing, including historical perspectives and current scope of practice. Psychiatric nursing involves the diagnosis and treatment of human responses to actual or potential health problems. The historical roots of psychiatry include early practices of curing the body of demon spirits, and later, acceptance of mental illness as a legitimate phenomenon that deserved specialized focus and attention. Peplau, in the mid-1900s, described the historical evolution of psychiatric–mental health nursing, including five eras, or phases:
1) Emergence of Psychiatric Mental Health Nursing (1773–1881);
2) Development of the Work Role of the Nurse in Mental Health Facilities (1882–1914); 3) Development of Undergraduate Psychiatric Nursing Education (1915–1935); 4) Development of Graduate Psychiatric Nursing Education (1936–1945); and 5) Development of Consultation and Research in Psychiatric–Mental Health Nursing (1946–1956). ANA Standards of Psychiatric–Mental Health Clinical Nursing Practice are reviewed, and education, career opportunities, and expanded roles of psychiatric nurses are discussed.

■ Chapter Outline

I. HISTORICAL DEVELOPMENT
   A. Prior to the fifth century, emotional disorders were believed to be an organic dysfunction of the brain, and clients were treated within healing environments that were conducive to improving symptoms in the mentally ill.
   B. During the Middle Ages, mental health treatment suffered setbacks: the mentally ill were considered to be possessed with demons, and to be incompetent and potentially dangerous; treatment often included cruel forms of torture.
   C. During the 18th century, reason and observation became the norm in treating the mentally ill, and individuals were treated in a more humane manner.

D. Peplau (1956) identified 5 phases of the development of psychiatric nursing:
   1. Phase 1 (1773–1881): Emergence of Psychiatric–Mental Health Nursing, during which Rush (1783) and Pinel (1792) made strides in studying and treating the mentally ill with compassion. Dorothea Lynde Dix (1870s) facilitated the emergence of state hospitals, with nursing to oversee care and operation of the wards.
   2. Phase 2 (1882–1914): Development of the work role of the Nurse in Psychiatric–Mental Health facilities, during which hospitals were established for the mentally ill, and the first training school for psychiatric nurses was established.
   3. Phase 3 (1915–1935): Development of Undergraduate Psychiatric–Mental Health Nursing Education; first psychiatric nurse graduated, journal articles and textbooks indicated a growing awareness of the knowledge of psychiatric nursing practice. Psychiatric classification system established (Kraepelin).
   4. Phase 4 (1936–1945): Development of Graduate Psychiatric–Mental Health Nursing Education; evolution of psychiatric nursing specialty, including graduate education curriculum guidelines.
   5. Phase 5 (1946–1956): Development of Consultation and Research in Psychiatric Mental–Health Nursing Practice; Mental Health Act (1946) set up funding for graduate nursing programs to prepare psychiatric clinical nurse specialists. NLN formed (1956), stressed that interest in psychiatric nursing should be stimulated to facilitate research, prevention, and cure for mental illnesses.
   6. Developments since 1956: Phenothiazines developed; Community Mental Health Act (1963) authorized funding for community health centers providing public treatment. 1990s known as the "Decade of the Brain" for focusing on biologic aspects of mental illness.

II. STANDARDS OF PSYCHIATRIC–MENTAL HEALTH CLINICAL NURSING PRACTICE
   A. *Standards of Psychiatric Mental Health Nursing Practice* (1982) developed by ANA.
   B. *Standards of Care and Standards of Professional Performance* (2000) developed by ANA.

III. PSYCHIATRIC–MENTAL HEALTH NURSING TODAY

    A. Education: Multiple programs are available to prepare psychiatric nurses at the generalist and specialist levels. Baccalaureate degrees provide theoretical, classroom, and clinical experiences. Master's degrees are available for clinical nurse specialist or nurse practitioner training.

    B. Career Opportunities: Opportunities for specialization, such as nurse liaison, private practice, psychotherapy, long-term care facilities, and mobile units.

    C. Expanded Role of Nurses: Certifications (such as in managed care nursing), privileges (such as admitting privileges), and forensic nursing are growing specialty roles.

KEY WORDS

Certification	Phenothiazines
Classification system in psychiatry	Privileging
Clinical Nurse Specialist	Psychiatric nurse practitioner
Community Mental Health Act	Standards of Care
Decade of the Brain	Standards of Practice
Forensic nursing	Standards of Professional Performance
Humane treatment	State mental hospitals
Peplau's five phases of psychiatric nursing	Therapeutic role of the psychiatric nurse

■ Classroom Teaching Strategies

1. Prior to class, ask students to interview a psychiatric nurse in their clinical setting, obtaining level of education, specialization, and psychiatric nursing role. Have students bring their findings back to the class for discussion of the variety of roles and educational paths that can be taken by psychiatric mental health nurses.

2. Divide the class into five groups, assigning each group one of Peplau's 5 Stages of Psychiatric Nursing Development. Instruct each group to act out the major events that occurred in the time period of their particular stage of nursing development, including key people and events, and their importance.

3. Have students construct a time line, beginning with the 5th century B.C., and include major events, individuals, and developments in the field of psychiatry, treatment of the mentally ill, and psychiatric–mental health nursing.

4. Provide students with or instruct students to obtain a copy of the Standards of Professional Performance. Ask each student to give an example of one of the Standards, including role definition, description of

a sample role activity, and the importance of that Standard in delivering psychiatric–mental health care.

5. Prior to class, assign students or groups of students to a prominent figure in the historical development of psychiatry. Allow class time for students to present a "historical snapshot" of this individual, including his or her philosophy and contribution to psychiatric–mental health practice. Examples include Hippocrates, Aristotle, Galen, Peplau, Rush, Pinel, Weyer, Kirkbridge, Dix, May, Beers, Kraepelin, Freud, Bleuler, Adler, Jung, Richards, and Bailey.

IV. AGREEMENT AMONG NURSING THEORISTS

There are many areas of agreement among theorists, including the concept that theories provide descriptions of nursing, offer a common language, need to be holistic, and provide frameworks for nurses in meeting client needs.

KEY WORDS

Behavioral responses to stress
Conceptual framework
Energy fields
Human adaptation
Human becoming
Interaction-oriented

Interpersonal relationships
Need-oriented
Nursing theory
Outcome-oriented
Self-care deficit
Systems-oriented theory

■ Classroom Teaching Strategies

1. Ask students individually, or in groups, to prepare a 15-minute presentation on a theorist of their choice, providing major theoretical concepts, nursing roles, and implications for practice, including an example.

2. Provide a vignette for students about a client and a functional difficulty, such as an individual with schizophrenia who is having trouble completing daily hygiene practices (bathing, brushing teeth, dressing). Ask students to discuss how the psychiatric nurse would intervene with this client, using each theorist's framework. Use the discussion period to illustrate differences between theorists' philosophies of client–nurse interaction, and differences in clinical approaches that arise from various theoretical viewpoints.

3. Divide students into three groups. Using need-oriented, outcome-oriented, and interaction-oriented frameworks, ask students to develop a plan of care for a depressed client with a focus on one of the three orientations.

4. Provide all students in the class with the same vignette: for example, a 30-year-old woman, married mother of two, who is admitted for depression. Divide the class into four groups, and assign each group one of Peplau's stages of the nurse–client relationship (orientation, identification, exploitation, resolution). Have each group act out an exchange between the nurse and client, given the particular stage of the relationship that is being portrayed. Discuss the progression through the four stages during the nurse–client relationship, using student portrayals as examples.

5. Ask students to write down an area of potential functional difficulty that is commonly experienced by psychiatric–mental health clients, and to develop an intervention based on a theorist of their choice. Have students share in class what they have developed, and use as a discussion forum about nursing theory and its application to clinical practice.

CHAPTER 4

Cultural and Ethnic Issues

■ Chapter Summary

Culture is a broad term referring to a set of shared beliefs, values, behavioral norms, and practices that are common to a group of people sharing a common identity and language. One's cultural background can shape decision making and behaviors surrounding health care. An ethnic group, or ethnicity, describes people within a larger social system whose members have common ancestral, racial, physical, or national characteristics, and who share cultural symbols such as language, lifestyles, and religion. Nurses must demonstrate sensitivity and respect for the individual client's unique beliefs, norms, values, and health practices when working with clients within the context of their cultural background. In the U.S., members of diverse ethnic groups do not utilize mental health care to the same extent as do members of the dominant European white middle class. Reasons for this include such issues as different languages, belief systems, values, and levels of health care coverage and economic status. The manner in which individuals perceive mental illness has a significant impact on their acceptance and use of psychiatric services. For example, some cultures see mental illness as a spiritual concern, and others view it as a lack of balance or harmony with the natural environment and with the body.

Ethnopharmacology is the study of how ethnicity affects drug metabolism. Ethnicity plays a role in the efficacy of psychoactive medications as well as the incidence of side effects.

■ Chapter Outline

I. CULTURE AND NURSING

    A. Definitions

        Culture is a broad term referring to a set of shared beliefs, values, behavioral norms, and practices that are common to a group of people sharing a common identity and language. One's cultural background can shape decision making and behaviors surrounding health care. An ethnic group, or ethnicity, describes people within a larger social system whose members have common ancestral, racial, physical, or national characteristics, and who share cultural symbols such as language, lifestyles, and religion. The tendency to believe that one's own way of thinking, believing, and behaving is superior to that of others is called *ethnocentrism*. Stereotyping occurs when one makes judgments or generalizations about members of a particular ethnic group without knowing that individual person. It is important for nurses to have awareness of their own and their client's cultural orientation when approaching the client's health care needs.

B. Culturally Congruent Nursing Care
Leininger (1991) developed a model using the concepts of worldview, social structure, language, ethnohistory, environmental context, and generic (folk) and professional systems to provide a comprehensive view of influences in cultural care and well-being. She proposed three culturally congruent nursing care modes: 1) cultural care preservation/maintenance; 2) cultural care accommodation and/or negotiation; and 3) cultural care repatterning/restructuring. Nurses must demonstrate sensitivity and respect for the individual client's unique beliefs, norms, values, and health practices when working with clients within the context of their cultural background.

II. POPULATION GROUPS
The federal government divides the population into five panethnic groups: 1) white; 2) black or African American; 3) Hispanic; 4) Asian/Pacific Islander; and 5) American Indian/Alaska Native. Nurses should ask clients what cultural group they identify with in order to avoid making assumptions about ethnicity.

III. USE OF MENTAL HEALTH SERVICES BY ETHNIC GROUPS
In the U.S. members of diverse ethnic groups do not utilize mental health care to the same extent as do members of the dominant European white middle class. Reasons for this include such issues as different languages, belief systems, values, and levels of health care coverage and economic status.

Nature of the Mental Health System: The U.S. mental health system was not designed to respond to the cultural and linguistic needs presented by individuals with diverse ethnicities. This fact, coupled with the differences that exist between providers' and clients' values, beliefs, health practices, and language, contributes to the difficulty in delivering mental health services to multicultural groups.

Socioeconomic Status of Ethnic Groups: According to statistics, many racial and ethnic groups have limited financial resources, and there is a correlation between lower socioeconomic status (i.e., income, education, occupation) and mental illness. Many people from diverse cultures in the U.S. lack adequate health insurance and/or are affected significantly by poverty. The psychiatric nurse encounters clients with multiple, complex problems related to the effect of poverty or to the fact that the cost of psychiatric care is not provided for in various insurance plans or is unaffordable to many families.

IV. CULTURAL PERCEPTIONS OF MENTAL ILLNESS
AND NURSING IMPLICATIONS
The manner in which individuals perceive mental illness has a significant impact on their acceptance and use of psychiatric services.

A. Mental Illness as Spiritual Concern: Some ethnic groups believe that mental illness is related to spirituality. The psychiatric nurse must be sensitive and responsive to individuals who may wish to integrate spiritual rituals into their prescribed plan of care.

B. Mental Illness as Imbalance or Disharmony in Nature: In some Native American cultures, mental illness is seen as a sign of imbalance with the rest of the natural world as well as in the human body. The nurse must provide culturally congruent care by seeking to understand and to intervene effectively with the client whose belief system focuses on mental illness as a lack of harmony with oneself and the world.

V. CULTURAL EXPRESSIONS OF MENTAL ILLNESS
AND NURSING IMPLICATIONS
The expression of mental illness symptoms and the way in which they are perceived vary widely between cultural groups. In many ethnic groups, there is no distinction among physical, mental, and spiritual illness. *Culture-bound syndrome* is a term used to signify recurrent locality-specific patterns of aberrant behavior and troubling symptoms that appear to fall outside conventional Western psychiatric diagnostic categories. The nurse should be aware that individuals from diverse ethnic groups may describe troubling experiences in terms of physical problems or specific culture-bound syndromes.

VI. PSYCHIATRIC NURSING OF ETHNIC GROUPS

A. Ethnopharmacologic Considerations: *Ethnopharmacology* is the study of how ethnicity affects drug metabolism. Ethnicity plays a role in the efficacy of psychoactive medications as well as the incidence of side effects.
Nursing Implications: The psychiatric nurse must collect ongoing data related to dosage and the incidence of side effects of medications in diverse cultural groups. Communication and collaboration with the physician is a key element in this approach to culturally sensitive care. In addition, teaching the client and family about the medications, nutrition, diet, and the use of herbal

and homeopathic remedies is critical to provide quality care to clients from a variety of cultural backgrounds.

B. Role of Family: The definition of what constitutes a family differs by ethnic group, as do roles assumed by different family members. Often members of diverse ethnic groups will not seek psychiatric treatment until exhausting the supports provided by family and community, and then when the client seeks assistance, the family members expect to be involved in the care.

Nursing Implications: Initial nursing assessment must include an evaluation of the members and roles of the client's family. Family members need to be included in treatment planning and teaching. A psychoeducational approach may be helpful in this situation, in which the nurse educates the family about the illness and offers supportive understanding about the family experience.

C. Role of Healers: Most ethnic cultures have traditional healers who speak the native tongue of the client and will intervene with mental health problems.

Nursing Implications: The psychiatric nurse must ask clients about their of healers during their assessment process, and may need to include the healer in the individual's multidisciplinary treatment team.

D. Role of Translators: Communication is vital to the delivery of psychiatric services, and thus many clients who are non-English-speaking may require a translator or interpreter. Privacy and confidentiality issues may affect the selection of the translator, and this choice must be made carefully.

Nursing Implications: If a translator is used, the nurse should speak directly to the client and use eye contact that is culturally congruent, should not interrupt the client and translator or use medical jargon, and should ask the client's permission to discuss emotionally charged topics.

VII. THE NURSING PROCESS

A. Assessment: Cultural assessment is an important part of the initial data collection for a nursing history, and should include assessment around concepts such as: 1) culture or ethnic group that the client identifies with; 2) family and support networks; 3) religious and spiritual practices; and 4) use of alternative therapies.

B. Nursing Diagnoses and Outcome Identification: The nurse analyzes any cultural data and determines how nursing care can preserve/maintain practices that are important to the client. Client outcomes that are relevant to the diagnosis and are realistic for the client's unique situation are identified.

C. Implementation: Implementations that are specific to cultural considerations include those that enable the nurse to do the following:
   1. Establish a trusting relationship
   2. Communicate with client and family
   3. Incorporate cultural beliefs

D. Evaluation: Nursing care is evaluated to determine that respect and understanding of the ethnically diverse client and family have been demonstrated. Client and family expression of satisfaction with nursing care is important and is the final measure of success of incorporating culturally appropriate nursing interventions.

KEY WORDS

Culturally congruent nursing care
Culture
Culture-bound syndrome
Ethnocentrism

Ethnopharmacology
Stereotyping
Subculture
Traditional healer

■ Classroom Teaching Strategies

1. Ask each student to identify one activity, issue, or event that he or she can associate with his or her own cultural background. Examples would include special holidays, foods, or ritual practices. Have students share their examples with the class.

2. Provide a clinical scenario of a client who is from a specific culture (Asian, African American, Latino, Spanish, for example) who comes into the Emergency Department with his extended family members. Ask students to divide into four groups. Each group is responsible for developing a plan for the following nursing assessment areas:
1) Assessment; 2) Nursing Diagnosis and Outcome Identification;
3) Implementation; and 4) Evaluation. Group 1 (Assessment) presents their assessment data, and Group 2 gets 10 minutes to develop a Nursing Diagnosis and Outcome Identification based on the assessment. Following Group 2's presentation, Group 3 (Implementation) would have 10 minutes to develop a plan; and following that group's presentation, Group 4 would discuss evaluation in connection with the plan that was presented. Use the steps as a springboard for discussion of multicultural issues in psychiatry.

3. Discuss with the class why different ethnic groups have varying degrees of response to psychotropic medications. Develop a nursing care plan based on this discussion.

4. Write each of the culture-bound syndromes on index cards. Pass out to groups of students in the classroom. Ask each group to communicate to

the class, in a culturally sensitive way and using creativity and multi-media, the particular syndrome and nursing responses to the client exhibiting these syndromes. Use the presentations as a discussion point for nursing assessment and intervention in a multicultural context.

5. Divide the class into groups, assigning each group to one psychotropic agent. Have students discuss potential clinical findings, psychopharmacology, and nursing care issues surrounding the psychotropic agent in diverse cultural groups.

CHAPTER 5

Ethical and Legal Issues

■ Chapter Summary

This chapter reviews concepts of ethics and legal issues in psychiatric nursing. *Ethics* is the study of values or value-laden decisions that conform to the moral standards of a group or of a profession. Psychiatric nurses are guided by the *ANA Code of Ethics for Nurses,* which includes the principles of the client's rights to autonomy, beneficence, justice or fair treatment, and veracity or truth regarding the client's condition and treatment. In recent decades, legal issues for nursing have emerged as an important area for study. Issues such as malpractice (the negligent conduct of a person acting within his or her professional capacity), confidentiality (the nondisclosure of private information related by one individual to another, such as from client to nurse), and privacy (the right to be left alone and free from intrusion or control) have been challenged in the legal system. Psychiatric hospitalizations, which can be voluntary or involuntary, are guided by the Bill of Rights for Psychiatric–Mental Health Clients. The psychiatric nurse must have adequate knowledge of both the law and of clients' rights to provide safe, effective care. Forensic psychiatry is an emerging specialty area in which mental health professionals are called upon to provide various types of consultation regarding a wide range of civil, criminal, and administrative proceedings. The forensic nursing role varies according to legal status of the client, treatment setting, and *ANA Standards for Practice in the Correctional Facility.*

■ Chapter Outline

I. ETHICS IN NURSING

    A. *Ethics* is a branch of philosophy that refers to the study of values or values-laden decisions that conform to moral standards of a group or a profession (Kelly, 1998). The ANA, in 1950, developed a code of ethics for nursing that is guided by four principles:

        1. The right to autonomy

        2. The right to beneficence (doing good) by the nurse

        3. The right to justice or fair treatment, and

4. The right to veracity or the truth regarding the client's condition and treatment (ANA, 1985).

B. Model of Ethical Nursing Care: Chally and Loriz (1998) developed a six-step ethical model for nursing decision-making:
   1. Clarify the ethical dilemma.
   2. Gather additional data.
   3. Identify options.
   4. Make a decision.
   5. Act, or carry out the decision.
   6. Evaluate the impact of the decision.

II. LEGAL ISSUES IN NURSING

The role of the nurse has changed significantly in recent decades, and nurses are subject to the scrutiny of federal and state regulations.

A. *Malpractice* is defined as the negligent conduct of a person acting within his or her professional capacity (Calloway, 1986). Four elements must be present for conduct to be considered negligent: 1) failure to act in an acceptable way; 2) failure to conform to the standard of care; 3) approximate cause, or the injury must be closely connected to the professional's conduct; and 4) the occurrence of actual damage. Examples of malpractice suits that have been brought against nurses include cases that involve: failure to follow physician's orders, medication errors, improper use of equipment, failure to remove foreign objects, failure to provide adequate monitoring, failure to communicate, assault and battery, defamation, and false imprisonment. The psychiatric nurse's knowledge of both the law and of the bill of rights for psychiatric clients reduces the risk of malpractice litigation.
   1. Confidentiality and Privacy: Breaches to confidentiality and privacy have become increasingly common due to the use of newer technologies (computers, e-mail, etc.). *Confidentiality* is the nondisclosure of private information related by one individual to another, such as from client to nurse. *Privacy* is defined as the right to be left alone and free from intrusion or control.
   2. Duty to Warn: The duty to warn an intended victim of a client's intent to harm takes precedence over the duty to protect a client's confidentiality. The *Tarasoff* decision reshaped the configuration of mental health practice and altered the relationship between clinicians and public authorities by stating that "the protective privilege ends where public peril begins."

B. Bill of Rights for Psychiatric–Mental Health Clients: The Mental Health Systems Act (1980) established the patient's bill of rights, which includes the rights to: 1) receive treatment; 2) refuse treatment; 3) a probable cause hearing within 3 court days of

involuntary admission; 4) privacy and confidentiality;
5) communicate freely with others; 6) personal privileges;
7) maintain one's civil rights; 8) religious freedom and education;
9) maintain respect, dignity, and personal identity; 10) maintain
personal safety and assert grievances; 11) transfer and continuity of
care; 12) access to own records; 13) explanation of costs and
services; and 14) aftercare.

C. Psychiatric Hospitalization: The type of psychiatric admission
depends on the mental status and presenting clinical symptoms of
the client. Clients may be admitted as an emergency or scheduled
visit, and psychiatric admissions can be classified as either
voluntary or involuntary. Involuntary patients who are a threat to
themselves or others may be admitted and detained for 72 hours in
the following situations: the person is mentally ill and has refused
voluntary examination after its purpose was explained, the person
is likely to suffer neglect if care is withheld, and there is danger that
the person will harm himself or others in the near future. Following
a 72-hour involuntary hold, a client may sign a voluntary consent
for treatment. If examination by two psychiatrists reveals the need
for continued treatment, a court hearing is required to extend
hospitalization. If the need for continued care is not established, the
client may be discharged without further care. Hospitalization of
minors is guided by individual state laws regarding their age and
legal rights.

D. Long-Term Care Facilities: Based on the Omnibus Reconciliation
Act (1987), a long-term care facility may not admit any new
resident needing active treatment for mental illness or mental
retardation. However, some long-term care facilities are willing to
admit psychiatric clients if they are stabilized and followed by a
psychiatrist or psychiatric nurse practitioner.

III. FORENSIC PSYCHIATRY
Forensic psychiatry is an emerging specialty area in which mental health
professionals are called upon to provide various types of consultation
regarding a wide range of civil, criminal, and administrative proceedings.
This includes the evaluation of an individual's competency and mental
condition at the time of an alleged crime.
    Role of the Forensic Nurse: The forensic nursing role varies
according to legal status of the client, treatment setting, and *ANA
Standards for Practice in the Correctional Facility*. The forensic nurse
may be called as an expert witness; the likelihood of this depends upon
the nurse's level of education, clinical training, licensure, specialty
board certification, experience, and reputation. The forensic nurse must
adhere to principles of honesty, strive for objectivity, and maintain
professional skills, interest, and empathy.

needs while developing a therapeutic plan of care. The continuum of care may continue in, for example, subacute care units, transitional care units, assisted-living or skilled nursing facilities, or adult day care, or may be part of home health care.

II. SUBACUTE CARE UNITS
Subacute care units, generally located within long-term care facilities, provide time-limited, goal-oriented care for clients who do not meet the criteria for continued hospitalization.

III. LONG-TERM CARE FACILITIES
The long-term care environment is rapidly changing due to the establishment of subacute and rehabilitation units within long-term care facilities. The clients most in need of admission to long-term care facilities are often those who also have the greatest need for psychiatric services.

IV. COMMUNITY MENTAL HEALTH
A. Description of Community Mental Health: Community mental health is the comprehensive psychiatric–mental health care of clients within their community of residence, with the goal of providing multidisciplinary, innovative treatment approaches. Five beliefs underlie this approach to treatment (Miller, 1981):
   1. Involvement and concern with the total community population
   2. Emphasis on primary prevention
   3. Orientation toward social treatment goals
   4. Comprehensive continuity of care
   5. Belief that community mental health should involve total citizen participation in need determination, policy establishment, service delivery, and evaluation of programs.
B. History of Community Mental Health
   The move toward community mental health, considered to be the third revolution in psychiatry (following the mental hygiene movement in 1908 and the development of psychopharmacology in the 1950s), gained prominence in the early 1960s. The National Mental Health Act provided funding for states to develop mental health programs outside of state psychiatric hospitals. States began the massive process of "deinstitutionalization," moving chronically mentally ill clients from state psychiatric hospitals back to their homes or to community-supervised facilities. The positive and negative effects of deinstitutionalization continue to significantly affect the field of community mental health.
C. Concepts of Community Mental Health
   Eight fundamental concepts provide the foundation for community mental health (Panzetta, 1985):

1. Use of a multidisciplinary team
2. The prevention of mental illness
3. Early detection and treatment
4. A comprehensive, multifaceted treatment program
5. Continuity of care
6. Group and family therapy
7. Environmental and social support and intervention
8. Community participation, support, and control
   Community mental health should be based on identified needs of deinstitutionalized individuals with specific psychiatric disorders, such as schizophrenia, bipolar disorder, or depression.

D. Types of Community Health Services
   1. Psychiatric Emergency Care: These services are designed to provide accessible crisis intervention, prevent unnecessary hospitalization, and decrease chronicity and dependence on institutional care.
   2. Day Treatment Programs: Usually 30- to 90-day programs that operate for 6 to 8 hours per day, 5 days a week, day treatment programs are designed to reduce hospitalization, decrease and stabilize psychiatric symptoms, provide successful work experiences, and in general facilitate the client's overall social functioning within the community.
   3. Residential Programs: One of the leading areas of program expansion in the care of the psychiatric client, residential care programs include: a) group homes; b) personal care homes; c) foster homes, d) satellite housing; and e) independent living. These programs have been found to be particularly effective with the chronically mentally ill client.
   4. Home Care: Visiting nurse home care in psychiatry, often delivered to the elderly, chronically mentally ill and clients in need of crisis intervention and short-term psychotherapy, is designed to provide comprehensive care, ongoing interdisciplinary collaboration, and accountability to client and community for the client who is homebound.
   5. Aftercare and Rehabilitation: Provided within the context of a community mental health center for the client who has been recently discharged from the hospital, aftercare and rehabilitation programs include services such as medication, individual and family therapy, crisis intervention, social skills training, medical care, and vocational training.

E. Role of the Community Mental Health Nurse
   Nurses play a major role in the provision of quality services to the psychiatric client in the community. Community mental health nurses, working within the ANA *Standards of Community Health Nursing*, provide counseling, support, and coordination of care and

health teaching. This role is comprehensive and challenging, requiring adaptability and flexibility.

V. THE CONTINUUM OF CARE IN THE 21ST CENTURY

A health care revolution is occurring on the World Wide Web, and mental health care providers and consumers are venturing into more direct therapeutic resources on the Internet. Chat rooms, educational resources, medication information, and even cybertherapy are all newly developing web-based resources that often can benefit persons who do not qualify for therapeutic intervention but are motivated for treatment. Another emerging practice setting is within the primary care setting, where about 25% of all clients have the diagnosis of mood disorder and are treated by the primary care clinician. In this setting, the nurse practitioner has the opportunity to provide consultation, diagnostic evaluation, psychotherapy, and the evaluation and management of psychotropic medication.

KEY WORDS

ANA Standards of Community Health Nursing
Case management
Community-based care
Community mental health
Cybertherapy

Deinstitutionalization
Managed care
Psychiatric nurse case manager
Psychiatric nurse practitioner
Utilization review

■ Classroom Teaching Strategies

1. Assign three groups of students to the following: a) Acute inpatient psychiatric hospitalization, b) a psychiatric subacute care unit, and c) long-term care facility. Describe a patient with schizophrenia who would be treated in each setting. Have each group describe: a) patient care that would be delivered in this setting; b) potential psychiatric–mental health nursing roles within the setting; and c) outcomes of psychiatric care that would be expected upon discharge from this setting. Use these descriptions to discuss the continuum of care in the psychiatric–mental health field.

2. Ask students to outline major ideological beliefs influencing community mental health, and to give examples of each.

3. Have students prepare a timeline of major events that have had an impact on the development of community mental health in psychiatry, and describe these events in terms of actual services that can be delivered to clients with mental illness.

4. Divide the class in half, and hold a debate about the positive versus negative effects of the deinstitutionalization movement in psychiatry.

5. Assign students to go on the Internet and locate at least one example of web-based psychiatric treatment or education. Encourage students to find the most creative or unusual types of websites that they can, and to discuss the pros and cons of these kinds of offerings for individuals and their families who may be experiencing symptoms of mental illness.

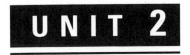
UNIT 2

Components of the Nurse-Client Relationship

CHAPTER 7

Assessment of Psychiatric–Mental Health Clients

■ Chapter Summary

The nursing process is a six-step problem-solving approach to nursing that also serves as an organizational framework for the practice of nursing. The six steps are: 1) Assessment; 2) Diagnosis; 3) Outcome Identification; 4) Planning; 5) Implementation; and 6) Evaluation. This chapter focuses on the first of the six steps: Assessment. The assessment phase includes collecting data about a person, family, or group by the methods of observing, examining, and interviewing. Objective data (information obtained verbally, by inspection, palpation, percussion, and auscultation) and subjective data (information that is spontaneously provided during direct questioning or during the health history) are gathered. The culturally competent nurse demonstrates sensitivity, knowledge, and skills while assessing culturally diverse groups of clients. Assessment includes gathering information about the following areas: appearance; affect, or emotional state; behavior, attitude, and coping patterns; communication and social skills; content of thought; orientation, memory, intellectual ability, insight; spirituality; sexuality; and neurovegetative changes. The psychiatric nurse must adequately, concisely, and completely document clinical findings from the comprehensive assessment in order to most effectively plan for the treatment and disposition of clients.

■ Chapter Outline

I. CLIENT ASSESSMENT

The assessment phase of the nursing process includes collecting data about a person, family, or group by the methods of observing, examining, and interviewing. Objective data (information obtained verbally, by inspection, palpation, percussion, and auscultation) and subjective data (information that is spontaneously provided during direct questioning or during the health history) are gathered.

A. Types of Assessment

Three kinds of assessment exist: 1) comprehensive assessment (data relating to the client's biological, psychological, cultural, spiritual, and social needs); 2) focused assessment (specific data regarding a particular client/family-identified problem); and 3) screening assessment (data from screening instruments used to evaluate a particular problem).

B. Cultural Competence During Assessment
Cultural competence is reflected in the nurse's sensitivity, knowledge, and skills in providing psychiatric care to culturally diverse groups of clients.

II. ASSESSMENT DATA COLLECTION

A. Appearance: General appearance includes physical characteristics, appearance, age, peculiarity of dress, cleanliness, and use of cosmetics, for example.

B. Affect, or Emotional State: *Affect* is the outward manifestation of a person's feelings, tone, or mood. Under ordinary circumstances, the person's affect varies according to the situation or subject under discussion.

C. Behavior, Attitude, and Coping Patterns: Behaviors and attitudes may vary as a result of coping patterns and types of supports available to the client.

D. Communication and Social Skills: The way in which clients talk provides data regarding thought processes and general psychopathologic disturbances. Impaired communication is described with the following terminology:
  1. Blocking: sudden stoppage in spontaneous stream of thinking or speaking for no apparent reason
  2. Circumstantiality: giving detail that delays meeting a goal or stating a point
  3. Flight of Ideas: overproductivity of talk and skipping from one topic to another
  4. Perseveration: persistent, repetitive expression of a single idea
  5. Verbigeration: meaningless repetition of incoherent words or sentences
  6. Neologism: a new word or combination of several words that are self-invented and not understood by others
  7. Mutism: refusal to speak

E. Content of Thought: Alterations in thought processes frequently seen in the psychiatric clinical setting include:
  1. Delusions: fixed, false beliefs not true to fact
  2. Hallucinations: sensory perceptions occurring in the absence of an external stimulus (can be auditory, visual, gustatory, or tactile)
  3. Depersonalization: feeling of unreality or strangeness about self or environment
  4. Obsessions: insistent thoughts that are usually regarded by the client as absurd and relatively meaningless

5. Compulsions: insistent, repetitive, intrusive, and unwanted urges to perform an act contrary to one's ordinary wishes or standards

F. Orientation: Orientation refers to the client's ability to grasp the significance of his or her environment, an existing situation, or the clearness of conscious processes.

G. Memory: Memory includes the ability to recall past experiences, both recent and long-term.

H. Intellectual Ability: The person's ability to use facts comprehensively reflects intellectual ability.

I. Insight Regarding Illness or Condition: Insight is defined as the person's self-understanding about the origin, nature, and mechanisms of one's attitudes and behaviors.

J. Spirituality: The client's beliefs, values, and religious culture are crucial components of a comprehensive examination.

K. Sexuality: This includes the client's sexual identity, function, and activities.

L. Neurovegetative Changes: Changes in psychophysiologic functions (sleep patterns, eating patterns, energy levels, sexual functioning, and bowel functioning, for example) provide critical information about symptoms that are often the target of psychotropic interventions. Although often neglected, information about the presence of sleep disturbances (such as insomnia) can be important. Primary insomnia refers to sleep problems that result from emotional or physical discomfort and are not due to the direct physiological effects of a substance or a general medical condition, while secondary insomnia is directly related to a psychiatric disorder.

III. DOCUMENTATION OF ASSESSMENT DATA

Information obtained by the psychiatric nurse during the assessment process is documented on the nursing admission/history form used by the specific psychiatric facility, and is reviewed by the interdisciplinary treatment team. Documentation should be: a) objective; b) descriptive; c) complete; d) legible; e) dated; f) logical; and g) signed. Nurses use various forms of documentation, such as SOAP (subjective data, objective data, assessment and plan of care) and DAP (objective and subjective data, assessment, and plan of care) notes. Nursing documentation should also reflect the effectiveness of treatment plans.

KEY WORDS

Blocking
Circumstantiality
Comprehensive assessment
Compulsions
Cultural competence
DAP notes
Delusions
Depersonalization
Flight of ideas
Focused assessment
Hallucinations
Insight

Mutism
Neologism
Neurovegetative changes
Nursing process
Obsessions
Orientation
Perseveration
Primary insomnia
Screening assessment
Secondary insomnia
SOAP notes
Verbigeration

■ Classroom Teaching Strategies

1. Show a clip from a popular film or TV movie that illustrates an individual who is emotionally upset (crying, laughing, labile mood, angry). Provide time during class for students to describe in detail the presentation of the client using the appropriate headings for assessment (appearance, affect or emotional state, mood, attitudes, and behaviors, etc.). Ask students to demonstrate how they might present this client to a multidisciplinary group of professionals.

2. Write symptoms of impaired communication on index cards (Blocking, Circumstantiality, Flight of Ideas, Perseveration, Verbigeration, Neologism, and Mutism). Divide students into pairs or groups of three. Give each group an index card, and have them creatively demonstrate the symptom, discussing its definition and associated behaviors.

3. Ask students to write down an example of each of the following types of hallucinations: auditory, visual, olfactory, tactile, and gustatory.

4. Have students discuss the differences between comprehensive, focused, and screening assessments, including their goals and purposes.

5. Ask students to list the criteria for documentation of assessment data (objective, descriptive, complete, legible, dated, logical, and signed) and to discuss the importance of such criteria in psychiatric mental health care.

CHAPTER 8

Nursing Diagnosis, Outcome Identification, Planning, Implementation, and Evaluation

■ Chapter Summary

The nursing process consists of six steps and uses a problem-solving approach. The previous chapter focused on the first step, assessment. This chapter focuses on the remaining five steps: nursing diagnosis; outcome identification; care planning; implementation, or nursing interventions; and evaluation of the client's response to interventions. Nursing diagnosis is a data-based clinical judgment that provides the basis for selecting interventions. Clinical nurse specialists and nurse practitioners in psychiatry use the DSM-IV-TR to make a psychiatric diagnosis when such a problem exists. Outcomes are measurable client-oriented goals that are expected consequences of a treatment or intervention. They drive the plan of care, which should always be individualized, is sometimes standardized, and the implementation of which is directed by a nursing theory. The evaluation of the care plan's effectiveness should be monitored and communicated by all members of the interdisciplinary health care team, including the client and family. As a result of this evaluation process, the care plan is maintained, modified, or totally revised. The nursing process is an ongoing, systematic series of actions, interactions, and transactions designed to promote optimal mental health in the client.

■ Chapter Outline

I. NURSING DIAGNOSIS

The nursing diagnosis is a statement of an existing or potential health problem that the nurse is both competent and licensed to treat. The psychiatric nurse analyzes the assessment data before determining a nursing diagnosis. Using the NANDA diagnostic system, nursing diagnosis is organized around nine human response patterns (exchanging, communicating, relating, valuing, choosing, moving, perceiving, knowing, and feeling), whereas the psychiatric–mental health nursing diagnostic system is organized around eight human response processes (activity, cognition, ecological, emotional, interpersonal, perception, physiologic, and valuation). Because integration of the NANDA and the psychiatric nursing models has not been completed, the psychiatric nursing community has agreed to use the NANDA classification until further integration has occurred.

Insurance companies require the use of a multiaxial system in psychiatric–mental health care known as the *Diagnostic and Statistical Manual of Mental Disorders,* 4th edition, text revision (DSM-IV-TR) published by the American Psychiatric Association (APA, 2000). The DSM-IV-TR presents structured decision trees to help the clinician understand the organization and hierarchical structure of the DSM-IV-TR classification.

II. OUTCOME IDENTIFICATION

Expected outcomes (the consequences of a treatment or an intervention) are measurable client-oriented goals that are realistic in relation to the client's present and potential capabilities, and they serve as a record of change in the client's health status.

III. PLANNING

The next phase of the nursing process is the development of a plan of care to guide therapeutic intervention and to achieve expected outcomes. Standardized care plans are often used in the clinical setting for specific nursing diagnoses, such as anxiety and fear. Managed care companies use such instruments to balance quality of care and cost containment.

IV. IMPLEMENTATION

The nurse uses various skills to implement the plan of care. Interventions for general psychiatric nursing practice, as well as clinical nurse specialty practice, are categorized according to the nurse's level of education and certification. Generalist interventions include nursing activities such as maintaining the therapeutic environment or milieu, psychobiologic interventions, health education, and case management. Specialist interventions include individual, group, family, and child therapy; pharmacologic agent prescription; and consultation with other health care providers.

V. EVALUATION

The evaluation phase focuses on the client's status, progress toward goal achievement, and ongoing reevaluation of the care plan. All members of the interdisciplinary health care team, including the client and family, should be encouraged to provide feedback regarding the effectiveness of the plan of care. As a result of this evaluation process, the care plan is maintained, modified, or totally revised.

KEY WORDS

Critical pathway

Decision tree

DSM-IV-TR

Expected outcome

Multiaxial system of diagnosis

NANDA diagnosis

Nursing diagnosis

Standardized care plan

■ Classroom Teaching Strategies

1. Provide the student with the following clinical scenario: Mr. B. is a 25-year-old African American male who presents to the inpatient unit for acute hospitalization. He is psychotic, mumbling that "people here are just out to get me!" and pacing up and down the hallway. He is disheveled, is wearing torn clothing, and smells of body odor. Ask students to: a) define two potential NANDA nursing diagnoses; b) develop at least two expected outcomes from the identified diagnoses; c) design two nursing interventions for each of the identified outcomes; and d) provide criteria for evaluation of the effectiveness of the identified nursing interventions.

2. Ask students to write one nursing diagnosis that might be made in the acute care hospital and to identify two expected outcomes, with nursing interventions and rationale.

3. Assign one of the following NANDA diagnoses to each group of students in class, and ask them to develop appropriate two short- and long-term expected outcomes for each:
   a. Anxiety, moderate level, related to physical condition and hospitalization as evidenced by tremulous voice, increased verbalization with pressured speech, and tremors of hands when speaking, and diaphoresis.
   b. Ineffective coping related to separation from family and home, change in physical status, and limited mobility.
   c. Disturbed sleep pattern related to anxiety secondary to physical illness as evidenced by the inability to fall asleep.
   d. Ineffective Sexuality Patterns related to fear and anxiety about sexual functioning secondary to physical illness.

4. Have students discuss why it may be difficult to develop a single nursing classification system in psychiatry, as evidenced by the NANDA and psychiatric nursing diagnostic classification systems.

5. Have students identify priorities for the first 24 hours of nursing care of a patient who is admitted to the inpatient setting for acute depression, accompanied by suicidal ideation.

CHAPTER 9

Therapeutic Communication and Relationships

■ Chapter Summary

Therapeutic relationships between client and nurse are established through communication and interaction and can be difficult and challenging. Communication involves interactions between the sender, the message, and the receiver. Both verbal and nonverbal methods of communication are powerful means to transmit messages and need to be the focus of attention in the client—nurse relationship. Therapeutic and social interactions are very different from one another, and each has unique qualities and techniques. The nurse uses therapeutic communication to help the client progress toward independence. Throughout the therapeutic relationship, it is important for the nurse to maintain confidentiality of the patient's clinical status in order to establish and maintain trust. The psychiatric nurse has many roles in the therapeutic relationship and uses techniques associated with three phases (orientation, working, and termination) to assist clients' movement through therapy.

■ Chapter Outline

I. COMMUNICATION
Communication involves three elements: the sender, the message, and the receiver.
A. Communication is a learned process and is influenced by many factors, including:
   1. Attitude: can be accepting, caring, prejudiced, judgmental, open- or closed-minded
   2. Sociocultural background: culture and heritage
   3. Past experiences: positive or negative experiences color one's ability to relate.
   4. Knowledge of subject matter: may increase person's security with topic
   5. Ability to relate to others: can occur naturally, or be learned with practice
   6. Interpersonal perceptions: using the senses during communication

7. Environmental factors: time, place, people present, noise level

B. Nonverbal Communication: People have less control over nonverbal behaviors, and they may reflect a more accurate picture of true feelings. Forms of nonverbal communication, with examples, in the psychiatric setting may include the following:
   1. Vocal cues: speech patterns, volume
   2. Gestures: movements with fingers, body, face that may show feelings of anxiety, insecurity, and genuineness, for example
   3. Physical appearance: grooming, clothing and dress, body size
   4. Distance or spatial territory: four zones in middle-class America: intimate, personal, social, and public
   5. Position or posture: sitting, slumped, standing rigidly
   6. Touch: touching another person
   7. Facial expressions: smiling, sadness, startled expression, blank stare

C. Effective Communication: is dependent on one's comfort zone with others. For better communication, broader comfort zones are helpful. Things that enable the nurse to establish broader comfort zones include:
   1. Know yourself.
   2. Be honest with your feelings.
   3. Be secure in your ability to relate to people.
   4. Be sensitive to the needs of others.
   5. Be consistent.
   6. Recognize symptoms of anxiety.
   7. Watch your nonverbal reactions.
   8. Use words carefully.
   9. Recognize differences.
   10. Recognize and evaluate your own actions and responses.

D. Ineffective Communication: Problems or stalls may occur during communication. Ineffective communication can be caused by some of the following:
   1. Failure to listen
   2. Conflicting verbal and nonverbal messages
   3. A judgmental attitude
   4. Misunderstanding because of multiple meanings of English words
   5. False reassurance
   6. Giving advice rather than encouraging self-confidence
   7. Disagreeing with or criticizing a person who is seeking support
   8. The inability to receive information because of a preoccupied or impaired thought process
   9. Changing the subject if one becomes uncomfortable with the topic

II. SOCIAL AND THERAPEUTIC INTERACTIONS
Social interactions occur daily with "small talk," greetings, and comments on the weather, for example. When interacting therapeutically, the nurse encourages the client to communicate his or her feelings.

A. Purtilo (1978) suggests the following approaches for participating in therapeutic interaction:
   1. Translate any technical information into layperson's terms.
   2. Clarify and restate instructions or information.
   3. Display a caring attitude.
   4. Be an effective listener.
   5. Do not overload the listener with information.

B. Confidentiality During Interactions: This is extremely important, because the client has a right to privacy. The nurse must maintain confidentiality and reassure the client that this will be upheld, except if the client threatens self-harm.

C. Interaction or Process Recording: A tool used to analyze nurse–client interactions. Usually includes verbal and nonverbal communication and may be done in many formats.

III. THE ONE-TO-ONE NURSE–CLIENT THERAPEUTIC RELATIONSHIP
An important goal of the psychiatric nurse is to develop a therapeutic relationship. *Transference* is a term used to describe the client's distortion of the nurse–client relationship, when the client relates to the nurse not based on personal attributes, but instead based on other interpersonal relationships in his or her environment. *Countertransference* is when the nurse responds unrealistically to the client.

A. Conditions Essential for a Therapeutic Relationship: Rogers (1961) listed eight essential conditions for establishing a therapeutic relationship:
   1. Empathy
   2. Respect
   3. Genuineness
   4. Self-disclosure
   5. Concreteness and specificity
   6. Confrontation
   7. Immediacy of relationship
   8. Self-exploration

B. Roles of the Psychiatric–Mental Health Nurse in a Therapeutic Relationship: Peplau (1952) described six subroles (each of which can be effective during different phases of the relationship) of the psychiatric nurse during a therapeutic relationship:
   1. Teacher

2. Mother surrogate
3. Technical nurse
4. Manager
5. Socializing agent
6. Counselor or nurse-therapist

C. Phases of a Therapeutic Relationship: One-to-one nurse–client therapeutic relationships can be divided into three phases:
  1. Initiating or Orienting Phase: Nurse becomes acquainted with client and sets the stage for the one-to-one relationship. Tasks include: build trust and rapport, privacy, establish communication that is acceptable to client and nurse, initiate a therapeutic contract, and assess client's strengths and weaknesses.
  2. Working Phase: Client begins to trust, relax, discuss feelings and goals, and focus on painful aspects of life. Tasks include: explore reality perceptions, develop positive coping behaviors, identify supports, enhance self-confidence, encourage verbalization, develop plan and goals, implement and evaluate plan, and promote client's independence.
  3. Termination Phase: When mutually agreed-upon goals are met, and separation occurs between client and nurse. Common goals met by termination phase include: provide self-care, demonstrate independence, recognize signs of illness, cope positively with negative experiences and feelings, and demonstrate emotional stability.

KEY WORDS

Client confidentiality
Countertransference
Nonverbal communication
Orientation phase
Personal comfort zone
Phases of therapeutic relationship

Process recording
Termination phase
Therapeutic relationship
Transference
Verbal communication
Working phase

■ Classroom Teaching Strategies

1. Divide the class into pairs. Distribute cards that have the following written on them: "Orientation Phase," "Working Phase," "Termination Phase" (you can make multiple cards depending on the number of students in your class). Ask each pair to demonstrate a nurse–client interaction that might occur at the phase listed on their card. Alternatively, ask each pair to discuss two tasks of the psychiatric nurse during the phase listed on their card.

2. Ask for three volunteers from class. Have two of them act out a role-play in which the psychiatric student nurse carries out "small talk" with a new client. Have the other student be the "recorder" and write the interaction down in column format on the board, leaving columns for "Verbal interaction," "Nonverbal behavior," "Student nurse's feelings," and "Ideas for more effective communication." Problem-solve with the class to fill in the columns on the board in relation to the role play.

3. Divide the class into halves, and have one half of the class demonstrate and discuss a "social" relationship; have the other half demonstrate and discuss a "therapeutic" relationship. Instruct students to highlight concepts that distinguish these types of relationships from each other.

4. Ask students to think about a relationship in which they are: 1) the client working with a professional; and 2) friends with someone. Have them write down their own personal feelings about each type of relationship, and some of the issues they face when interacting with the other person in that relationship. Focus on student perceptions of what is helpful behavior of the professional in the client–professional relationship, and make analogies to the role of the psychiatric nurse.

5. Ask students to list as many types of professional relationships as they can think of. Write students' ideas on the blackboard or overhead. Then, have students discuss and differentiate what might be different or the same about these relationships and the client–nurse relationship. Help students focus on aspects of professional relationships that are helpful to the client (such as trust, empathy, knowledge, etc.).

CHAPTER 10

The Therapeutic Milieu

■ Chapter Summary

Milieu therapy is socioenvironmental therapy in which the attitudes and behavior of the staff in a treatment service and client activities are determined by the client's emotional and interpersonal needs. The client's environment is organized to assist him or her to control problematic behavior, with the focus on social relationships and occupational and recreational activities. Psychiatric nurses often assume responsibility for managing and coordinating activities within the therapeutic milieu. Components that may be useful to facilitate client healing and growth within the context of the therapeutic milieu include such things as education, spirituality, personal and sleep hygiene, protective care, behavior therapies, and adjunctive or management therapy. It is important to frequently assess the therapeutic milieu. One instrument that has been used to evaluate milieu effectiveness is the Ward Atmosphere Scale (WAS), which is valuable in assessing a variety of inpatient and outpatient therapeutic settings.

■ Chapter Outline

I. DEVELOPMENT OF THE THERAPEUTIC MILIEU
Standards have been set forth by JCAHO for the development of therapeutic milieu treatment environments. These standards specify that the milieu should: be purposeful and planned for safety; provide testing grounds for new behaviors; have consistency with limits; encourage communication and group activities; provide respect and dignity to clients; convey an attitude of acceptance and optimism; and assess and evaluate client progress in treatment. Members of the psychiatric multidisciplinary team in the milieu include psychiatric nurses, nursing assistants, or technicians; psychiatrists; clinical psychologists; psychiatric social workers; other therapists, such as art and music therapists; chaplains; dietitians; and auxiliary personnel. The psychiatric nurse often has responsibility for the management and coordination of activities within the milieu.

II. COMPONENTS OF THE THERAPEUTIC MILIEU

Interventions in the therapeutic milieu that meet the basic needs of the client in the psychiatric setting include:

A. Education: client education can be accomplished by the psychiatric nurse through a variety of strategies, including such activities as: prioritizing the client's needs and daily foci; presenting specific information; using simple language; using different educational approaches; involving family and social supports; and educating and reinforcing information while providing care.

B. Spirituality: This is a feeling associated with a transcendent dimension, a manifestation of one's spiritual drive to create meaning in the world. Spiritual beliefs can affect recovery rate and attitudes toward treatment. Psychiatric nursing assessment and intervention should include spiritual assessment, and identification of barriers to client's spiritual needs.

C. Personal and Sleep Hygiene: *Activities of daily living* is a term used to describe the client's ability to feed, bathe, dress, and toilet himself or herself. Clients in the psychiatric setting often experience disturbances of sleep, for which various nursing interventions may be helpful. Psychopharmacologic sleep agents can also promote sleep.

D. Protective Care: Because the potential for violence is inherent in an inpatient psychiatric unit, the psychiatric nurse must be vigilant in assessing and intervening with escalating behavior. This may include the safe and flexible use of seclusion and restraints. Protective nursing care includes observation and care so the client does not injure himself or herself or others, or become injured when around other clients.

E. Behavior Therapy: Behavior therapy focuses on modifying behaviors by systematically manipulating the environment and variables that are connected with the dysfunctional behavior (APA, 1994). Behavior therapies (and a brief description of each) are interventions such as:

1. Behavior Modification and Systematic Desensitization: The use of rewards to reinforce desired behaviors is behavior modification. Desensitization is based on Pavlov's theory of conditioning, and emphasizes relaxation techniques that inhibit anxious responses.

2. Aversion Therapy: The use of unpleasant or noxious stimuli to change undesired behavior.

3. Cognitive Behavior Therapy: Using confrontation as a means of helping clients restructure irrational beliefs and behaviors.

4. Assertiveness Training: Teaching clients how to relate to others using frank, honest, direct expressions.

5. Implosive Therapy: This is also called flooding, and is the

opposite of systematic desensitization. The client is exposed to intense forms of anxiety-producing stimuli.

6. Limit Setting: This intervention involves providing a framework for the client to function in, which reduces anxiety and minimizes manipulation. The consequence of limit setting should not provide secondary gain or lower self-esteem.

F. Adjunctive or Management Therapy: These include therapies such as occupational, educational, art, music, psychodrama, recreational, play, speech, and nutritional therapy.

III. ASSESSMENT OF THE THERAPEUTIC MILIEU

The Ward Atmosphere Scale (WAS; Moos, 1974) is used to assess the effectiveness of the therapeutic milieu, and includes 10 subscale items that provide information about what actually exists and what should exist in the milieu. The instrument is appropriate for evaluating a wide variety of treatment environments, such as inpatient units and day treatment centers. Subscales of the WAS focus on the following elements: staff control of rules, schedules, and client behavior; program clarity; client involvement in the milieu; preparing the client for discharge; supportive atmosphere of clients; environmental spontaneity that allows free expression of feelings; promoting responsibility and self-direction; order and organization of the unit; and encouragement of verbalization by clients and channeling of feelings into appropriate behavior.

KEY WORDS

Adjunctive therapy	Milieu
Aversion therapy	Milieu therapy
Behavior therapy	Protective care
Cognitive behavior therapy	Systematic desensitization
Implosive therapy	Ward Atmosphere Scale
Limit setting	

■ Classroom Teaching Strategies

1. Ask students to take the Ward Atmosphere Scale (WAS) to their clinical site, complete the tool, and bring it back to class. Have students identify similarities and differences in their findings. Discuss the difficulties the students assessed, and facilitate a problem-solving session in which students make recommendations for what might improve the milieu.

2. Write the various forms of behavior therapy (behavior modification; systematic desensitization; aversion therapy; cognitive behavior therapy; assertiveness training; implosive therapy; and limit setting) on index cards, divide the class into groups, and provide one card per group. Ask

each group to briefly define the type of therapy, and using any creative method they wish, illustrate or describe the type of therapy with an example.

3. Ask students to come to the blackboard and to write down two examples for each of the following components of the therapeutic milieu: Education, Spirituality, Personal and Sleep Hygiene, Protective Care, Adjunctive or Management Therapy.

4. Have an open class discussion about treatment milieu, the definition, nursing interventions, and goals of using milieu therapy.

5. Have students compare the characteristics of a treatment milieu to that of a small community, and highlight goals for client learning that are related to social relationships and interpersonal interactions with the environment.

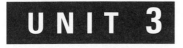
UNIT 3

Interactive Therapies

CHAPTER 11

Crisis Intervention

■ Chapter Summary

Most people exist in a state of equilibrium. Everyday life contains some degree of harmony in one's thoughts, feelings, wishes, and physical needs. Stress occurs when there is a serious interruption or disturbance in this harmony. Equilibrium may be disrupted and the individual may experience a state of emotional turmoil. When this occurs, one may be experiencing a crisis. Crises are often sudden, involve a failure of normal coping, are usually short in duration, and cause increased psychological vulnerability for the individual. Crises can be maturational (when one's lifestyle is continually subject to change, such as adolescence, marriage, or aging, for example) or situational (a particular, extraordinarily stressful event, such as an illness or accident, for example). Five phases of crisis have been identified: 1) precrisis; 2) impact; 3) crisis; 4) resolution; and 5) postcrisis. Crisis intervention is an active, temporary entry into an individual's life situation during a period of stress, the goals of which are to decrease emotional distress, to assist the client in organizing and mobilizing resources, and to return the client to a precrisis or higher level of functioning. Psychiatric nurse clinicians and nurse practitioners play key roles in assisting individuals and families through crises, and work using a variety of treatment approaches, such as individual, group, suicide intervention, and mental health center crisis intervention modalities.

■ Chapter Outline

I. CHARACTERISTICS OF A CRISIS
   A. Suddenness: A crisis usually occurs suddenly, and one is inadequately prepared to handle the event or situation.
   B. Failure of normal coping: There is a failure of normal coping mechanisms, and feelings of anxiety, fear, and helplessness may occur.
   C. Short in duration: A crisis is usually short-lived, lasting anywhere from 24 to 36 hours to 4 to 6 weeks.
   D. Increased psychological vulnerability: During a crisis, an individual

may demonstrate potentially self-injurious behaviors or, alternatively, may experience personal growth.

II. PHASES OF A CRISIS

A. Precrisis: A general state of equilibrium in which the person is able to cope with everyday stress.

B. Impact: A stressful event occurs that precipitates a crisis state.

C. Crisis: A time during which the person is confused, anxious, and disorganized because he or she feels helpless and normal coping mechanisms are not working.

D. Resolution: A time during which the individual regains control of emotions, handles the situation, and works toward a solution for the crisis.

E. Postcrisis: The resumption of normal living activities after living through a crisis.

III. CLASSIFICATION OF A CRISIS ACCORDING TO SEVERITY
Burgess and Baldwin (1981) described six types of crises based on the severity of the event.

A. Class 1: Dispositional crisis; when a problem needs immediate action

B. Class 2: Life transitional crisis; occurs during normal growth and development

C. Class 3: Crisis due to sudden, unexpected traumatic event

D. Class 4: Maturational crisis; developmental event during which stress is internal and involves psychosocial issues

E. Class 5: Pre-existing psychopathology; when depression or anxiety, for example, interfere with normal functioning

F. Class 6: Psychiatric emergencies; unpredictable or self-injurious behavior

IV. PARADIGM OF BALANCING FACTORS
Aguilera (1994) describes a paradigm of factors that enable a return to equilibrium: a) realistic perception of the event; b) adequate situational support; and c) adequate coping or defense mechanisms to help resolve the problem.

V. CRISIS INTERVENTION
Crisis intervention is an active, temporary entry into an individual's life situation during a period of stress. The client is encouraged to be active in all steps of the process. Crisis intervention can occur in a wide variety of settings and can be generic (focused on a particular type of crisis) or individual (stresses the present, immediate causes of the crisis)

in approach. Goals of crisis intervention are to:

A. Decrease emotional distress

B. Assist client in organizing and mobilizing resources

C. Return client to precrisis or higher level of functioning

VI. ROLE OF NURSE CLINICIAN OR NURSE PRACTITIONER DURING A CRISIS

Clinicians must understand the effects of severe stress on the average person. They become prepared to assist crisis victims through educational programs in crisis intervention techniques. Clinicians' attitudes may affect the outcome of the client's response. A multidisciplinary approach is optimal in facilitating crisis resolution.

A. Steps in Crisis Intervention

1. Assessment: Involves a) assessment of the degree of client's disruption. Crisis forensics is a specialized assessment of the dangerousness of the client's behavior toward self or others; b) assessment of the client's perception of the event, including the significance of the event in the client's life; c) formulating nursing diagnoses as foci for treatment.

2. Planning the Therapeutic Intervention: Client should be involved in planning for interventions that will be most helpful in working toward crisis resolution.

3. Implementing the Therapeutic Intervention: Depends on the pre-existing skills, creativity, and flexibility of the crisis worker and the rapidity of the person's response. A range of therapeutic techniques are used when performing crisis intervention.

4. Resolution with Anticipatory Planning and Evaluation: Reassessment must occur throughout the intervention to assure that the crisis intervention is reducing tension and anxiety. Reinforcement is important, and assistance is provided to formulate realistic plans for the future.

B. Crisis Intervention Modes

Individual crisis intervention is common. However, clients may choose to work within a group modality to resolve crises through use of the group process. A crisis group meets from 4 to 6 weeks, providing support, encouragement, and suggestions.

Family crisis counseling may also be beneficial, where the entire family comes for sessions for about 6 weeks. Suicide prevention and crisis intervention centers often include telephone hotlines, staffed by volunteers who have had intensive training in telephone interviewing and counseling and can give immediate assistance.

Mental health crisis intervention services are often hospital-based or tied to community mental health centers. Mobile crisis units may also be used, to provide services to clients who may not have access to health care centers.

C. Legal Aspects of Crisis Intervention

The National Crisis Prevention Institute (CPI) has trained many human service providers in the technique of nonviolent crisis intervention. The criteria and standards of care for a person providing crisis intervention state that the person who begins to intervene in a crisis must continue the intervention unless a more qualified person intervenes to relieve him or her. Discontinuing care constitutes abandonment. Negligence may be charged if a person is injured by the actions of a crisis worker.

KEY WORDS

Anticipatory planning
Balancing factors
Crisis
Crisis forensics
Crisis intervention
Crisis intervention training

Defenses or coping mechanisms
Maturational crisis
Situational crisis
Situational supports
Suicide prevention counseling

■ Classroom Teaching Strategies

1. Ask students to bring a newspaper clipping that reports a crisis situation. Have them identify what type of crisis is being reported (situational, maturational, dispositional, life transition, psychiatric emergency, for example), and how they might assess and intervene with the victims of the crisis.

2. Provide students with the following scenario: "A group of 10-year-old students traveling to a field trip were in a bus accident. Their bus was struck by a train. There were no injuries, but the children were very emotionally shaken. The group of children are brought to the gymnasium of the local elementary school for a discussion about the accident." Ask students to describe the type of crisis being portrayed, what types of reactions they might anticipate from students, and some techniques for how they might intervene in this situation. Use the exercise to emphasize the different treatment approaches and modalities (ie, group vs. individual) that can be useful in crisis intervention, and to highlight overall goals of crisis intervention.

3. Have students think about a school-related crisis they have experienced (for example, failing an exam, or a clinical experience that may have been difficult). Ask them to list some of their common feelings, thoughts, and reactions to the crisis. Have them plot a timeline to illustrate the process they went through to resolve the crisis, including time involved. Use the exercise to highlight the time frame of crises, the process of resolution and crisis intervention, and the benefits/drawbacks of having an objective

outsider who may help with crisis management vs. handling the crisis alone.

4. Have an open discussion about how people handle crisis: what are some of the common reactions and feelings, the process of going through and resolving crisis, differing ways that people cope with crisis (ie, alone vs. getting help), and outcomes that may be associated with different types of crisis management (ie, coming out of the crisis with a better self-understanding, or coming out of a crisis with a major depression, etc.). Identify coping techniques that facilitate positive outcomes.

5. Have a brainstorming session about every crisis that students can think of. Write them on the blackboard. Then, sort the crises out by type and level of severity, and put them into groups, discussing techniques that might be useful for that type of crisis (ie, maturational, situational, etc.).

CHAPTER 12

Individual Psychotherapy and Group Therapy

■ Chapter Summary

Psychotherapy is the treatment of emotional and personality problems using psychological means that rely on the client–therapist relationship as an important factor. Psychotherapy is a process in which the person who wants to relieve symptoms enters into a contract to interact in a prescribed way with the therapist, who provides individual or group therapy, depending on client needs. Only the certified specialist in psychiatric mental health nursing can perform psychotherapy, but it is important for the psychiatric nurse to understand these dynamics. *Counseling* is a form of supportive psychotherapy that can be done by the psychiatric nurse within the context of the nurse–client relationship.

There are many forms of psychotherapy, including individual and group modalities. Individual therapy focuses on the internal psychology of the individual person, and includes such modalities as: brief cognitive therapy, behavioral therapy, and brief interpersonal therapy. Group psychotherapy, an alternative modality, is based on the use of group dynamics to increase the individual's functional level. Yalom (1985) identified 11 factors that enable groups to be effective. There are different types of group therapy, and the therapist must be alert to the philosophical framework of the group, tasks and goals of the group, stages of group development, and the role of the therapist in different group modalities. More recent approaches to psychotherapy include Internet-based interactions, such as telepsychiatry or video phone psychotherapy, for example.

Freud first described the psychotherapeutic process as a treatment that uses the interpersonal experience between client and therapist as a therapeutic modality. Transference (client's unconscious assignment to the therapist of feelings originally associated with other important figures in early life) and countertransference (the therapist's emotional reaction to the client based on the therapist's unconscious needs and conflicts) are forces that may interfere with therapeutic interventions during the course of psychotherapy treatment. Sullivan (1953) described parataxis, or the presence of distorted perceptions or judgments exhibited by the client during therapy, as a result of earlier interpersonal experiences.

■ Chapter Outline

I. INDIVIDUAL PSYCHOTHERAPY

The psychotherapeutic process is designed to facilitate understanding and insight into factors that might be unknown to the client, and may be among the causes of the disturbance for which the client is seeking help. There are three phases of therapy: introductory, working, and termination. The goals of individual psychotherapy are to alleviate the client's pain, change character structure and strengthen the ego, facilitate maturation, and improve the client's ability to act appropriately. Ways in which individual psychotherapy works include: establishing a therapeutic relationship; providing an opportunity for tension release; improving insight; providing an opportunity to practice new skills; reinforcing appropriate behavior; and providing consistent emotional support. Managed care has had a significant effect on the practice of psychotherapy. Conventional, longer-term individual therapies of the past have been replaced by brief cognitive therapies.

A. Brief Cognitive Therapy: Uses a time-limited, goal-oriented, problem-solving, here-and-now approach. The therapist is active and works to help the person solve problems by exploring alternative behaviors.

B. Behavior Therapy: Focuses on the modification of overt symptoms without addressing the client's inner conflicts. The therapist uses limit-setting, promoting positive adaptive behaviors and assertiveness, and assisting the client in exploring new ways to adjust to the environment.

C. Brief Interpersonal Psychotherapy: a semistructured, psychodynamically time-limited model of psychotherapy designed to be used in a 3- to 4-month framework. The therapist reinforces the client's self-esteem, employs a goal-directed approach, reinforces and supports use of positive defense mechanisms and coping skills, and avoids transference and countertransference unless necessary.

II. GROUP PSYCHOTHERAPY

Group psychotherapy is a method of therapy based on exploring individual and intrapsychic structures and the group process. The use of groups has long been an effective treatment method for psychiatric problem resolution. Members from several of the psychiatric disciplines, such as nursing, social work, family counseling, and others, participate as group therapists. Groups can be valuable in encouraging members to use each other's assets to foster their own growth, to become more aware of self, to learn acceptable behaviors, and to improve communication.

A. Characteristics of Group Therapy
   Yalom (1985) identified 11 curative factors as essential components of group therapy:
   1. Installation of hope
   2. Universality
   3. Imparting of information
   4. Altruism
   5. The corrective recapitulation of the primary family group
   6. The development of socializing techniques
   7. Imitative behavior
   8. Interpersonal learning
   9. Group cohesiveness
   10. Catharsis
   11. Existential factors

B. Types of Therapy Groups
   There are different types of groups that make use of major theoretical frameworks. Open groups do not have boundaries, and members may come and go at different times. Closed groups have a set membership, a specific time frame, or both. Both open and closed types of groups are used in inpatient and outpatient treatment settings. Marram (1978) identified five models of group therapy:
   1. Support groups
   2. Re-education and remotivation groups
   3. Problem-solving therapy groups
   4. Insight without reconstruction groups
   5. Personality reconstruction groups

C. Establishing a Group
   The selection of group participants is influenced by personal treatment philosophy. Elements for consideration when establishing a group include size; diagnosis of members; age; gender; intellectual level; communication and social skills; motivation; and the environmental setting.

D. Stages of Group Development
   All therapy groups have three major stages: a beginning or orientation phase, a middle or working phase, and an ending or termination phase. The key issues involve dependency and interdependency. The therapist hopes that when members leave the group, they are more realistic in their self-perceptions, have increased self-esteem, are better able to problem-solve, and are more equipped to assume responsibility for their lives.

E. Role of the Nurse Therapist
   There are many opportunities for the nurse to assume the role of group leader, group therapist, or co-therapist. Major qualifications that the nurse should possess include: a) theoretical preparation;

b) supervised clinical experience; and c) personal experience as a group therapy member. The ANA recommends that nurse therapists have a master's degree in psychiatric nursing and should be certified as clinical nurse specialists. Three basic styles of group leadership are autocratic, democratic, and laissez-faire; the use of a particular style depends on the therapist's theoretical and personal style.

III. COUNSELING
   The psychiatric nurse uses different types of counseling interventions to help clients to regain and improve coping skills. Some of these include:
   A. Communication and interviewing techniques
   B. Problem-solving skills
   C. Crisis intervention
   D. Stress management
   E. Relaxation techniques
   F. Assertiveness training
   G. Conflict resolution
   H. Behavior modification

IV. ALTERNATIVE APPROACHES TO PSYCHOTHERAPY
   There are some alternative approaches to psychotherapy that are in use, many of which relate to the therapist's use of technology and the Internet. Examples include psychotherapy over the Internet, electronic consultation to primary care physicians, telepsychiatry or video equipment with computer software, and videophone psychotherapy. Other types of psychotherapy that have been successful include modified life review therapy, cognitive therapy, and insight-oriented therapy in treating elderly clients who are depressed. Cross-cultural therapy is becoming essential in our society, where ethnic subcultures continue to grow.

KEY WORDS

Behavioral therapy
Brief cognitive therapy
Brief interpersonal psychotherapy
Closed group
Counseling
Countertransference

Open group
Parataxis
Psychotherapy
Telepsychiatry
Transference
Yalom's 11 curative factors

■ Classroom Teaching Strategies

1. Have students divide into three groups. Assign each group to one of the following phases: a) beginning or orientation phase; b) middle or working phase; c) ending or termination. Ask each group to consider the phase of group interaction, and to prepare a brief summary of the following issues: the therapist's role and tasks during this phase, and overall client objectives of this phase. Have each group present their findings to the class. If time permits, encourage students to utilize role-plays or other creative means to illustrate the group phase on which they are reporting.

2. Have students think about the meaning of transference and countertransference. Facilitate a class discussion about the meaning of these terms, their definitions, and examples of each. If students have been in clinical situations in which they have had the opportunity to experience or observe these phenomena, ask them to provide clinical examples.

3. If possible, prepare and assign this task 1 week in advance, to allow students time to prepare. Divide the class into three groups, and assign each group to: 1) brief cognitive therapy; 2) behavior therapy; or 3) brief interpersonal psychotherapy. Have each group provide a brief description of this type of therapy; explain why it might be more effective than the other two types; and provide an example of a clinical situation in which this type of therapy would be most effective. Use student presentations to stimulate a discussion of the efficacy and uses of different therapy modalities.

4. Write Yalom's 11 curative factors on index cards, one per card. Shuffle and randomly pass out the cards in class. Ask students to define and give an example of the factor that they chose.

5. Ask students to compare and contrast group therapy with individual therapy, outlining the goals of each, benefits and drawbacks, and therapist roles for each modality.

CHAPTER 13

Couple and Family Therapy

■ Chapter Summary

Families have undergone many changes in the past 50 years. In the family setting, members learn how to relate to and communicate with others. The family also can influence personal development positively or negatively. Family functioning occurs on a continuum from healthy to dysfunctional. When a family has difficulty or is under stress and becomes dysfunctional, family therapy is a treatment modality that can help the family to gain insight into their problems and change family behaviors. There are different types of therapies that are helpful to families in crisis. Couple therapy is useful to resolve tension or conflict in relationships. Family therapy helps family members to understand their difficulties and to improve communication and functioning of individual members and the family as a whole. There are several approaches to family therapy, including: psychoanalytic, structural, interactional or strategic, social network or systemic, and behaviorist approaches. The approach used depends on the therapist's training and treatment philosophy. The clinical nurse specialist or nurse practitioner with a graduate degree in psychiatric nursing can function as a family therapist. Nurse therapists use a variety of techniques to assist families in healing, including such activities as conducting family assessments, participating in family education, and providing family therapy.

■ Chapter Outline

I. FAMILY LIFE CYCLE

The family is a developing system that must progress in a healthy way in order for children to develop properly. There are eight phases of family development that are predictable and successive (Duvall, 1977): 1) beginning families (no children); 2) early childbearing; 3) families with preschool children; 4) families with school-aged children; 5) families with teenagers; 6) launching-center families; 7) families of middle years; and 8) families in retirement and old age.

II. HEALTHY FUNCTIONING FAMILIES

Healthy families have specific characteristics that include the ability to communicate thoughts and feelings, and parental guidance that determines the functioning level of the total family. In the healthy family, no one member dominates or controls another. Instead, there is a respect for individual points of view and opinions of each member. Good communication patterns are paramount. Each family member should progress through certain stages of individual development, and ego boundaries should be clearly developed. Family members do not function totally independently from one another, but interact in a mutually interdependent way.

III. DYSFUNCTIONAL FAMILIES

Some healthy families may become dysfunctional during times of stress. In the dysfunctional family, there is no clear leadership, and the resulting confusion causes increased dependency and lack of individuation of members. Communication is not open, direct, or honest and is usually confusing to other family members. Children and adults may be performing roles that are inappropriate to their age, sex, or personality.

IV. CULTURALLY DIVERSE FAMILIES

It is imperative that the nurse therapist consider the culture of the family, including social life, political systems, language and traditions, religion, health beliefs and practices, and cultural norms. Doing so will help to avoid labeling a family as dysfunctional because of cultural differences.

V. HISTORY OF FAMILY THERAPY

Family therapy has its roots in the 1950s, when psychotherapists began looking at the pattern of relationships of individuals that corresponded with family problems. Bowen, Ackerman, Minuchin, Haley, and Satir were early family psychotherapists. They began changing their approach from treating only the individual to including the family to help increase therapeutic effectiveness. The family therapist sees the family as a system of relationships, any breakdown of which affects every family member. Individual, group, couple, or family therapy may be useful for members of a dysfunctional family.

VI. COUPLE THERAPY

Couple therapy is a way of resolving tension or conflict in a relationship. A couple's beliefs about love, intimacy, gender roles, sexuality, and marriage determine the nature and quality of their relationship. Chisholm (1996) describes three types of couples therapy: 1) marital relations therapy; 2) contextual therapy; and 3) object relations therapy. The goal of couple therapy is to change troublesome behavior and dysfunctional patterns in the couple. Brief couple therapy is based on understanding each partner's belief systems and how these systems interlock to influence lives and relationships. When beliefs are acted upon over time, they form themes or emotional issues that dominate a relationship, which can cause recurring conflicts.

VII. FAMILY THERAPY

Family therapy is a treatment in which family members gain insight into problems. Family therapy is different from individual therapy because it focuses on outside or external forces (vs. internal forces) that play a role in personality development and family members' behaviors. As a family works through problems in therapy, each member's role should become more clear, and the family can become more functional.

A. Types of Family Therapy

Jones (1980) described seven orientations to family therapy: 1) integrative approach; 2) psychoanalytic approach; 3) Bowen approach; 4) structural approach; 5) interactional or strategic approach; 6) social network or systemic approach; and 7) behaviorist approach. Each of these approaches has its own theoretical basis and techniques that are used by the therapist to promote family growth and healing during the therapeutic process.

B. Goals of Family Therapy

The therapist and family need to discuss together the problems that are bringing the family into therapy. It is important for the therapist and family to discuss and to understand how each member perceives the family's difficulties. The overriding goal of family therapy is to facilitate positive changes in the family.

C. Stages of Family Therapy

There are three main stages of family therapy:

1. Initial Interview: During the initial interview, the therapist works to assess and synthesize all the information the family has provided and to formulate ideas or interventions for bringing about positive changes in the family.

2. Intervention or Working Phase: During this phase, the therapist helps the family to accept and adjust to change, and identifies the strengths and problems of the family.

3. Termination Phase: This phase begins when the family has learned how to solve its own problems in a healthy manner, has developed its own internal support system, and has learned to communicate in a more open, honest, and direct way. Termination occurs when the original family problems or symptoms have been alleviated.

D. The Nurse-Therapist's Role in Family Therapy

The clinical nurse specialist or nurse practitioner with a graduate degree in psychiatric nursing can function in a variety of highly skilled roles, one of which is serving as a family therapist. Psychiatric nursing specialists utilize a variety of techniques to assist families in healing, including such activities as conducting family assessments, participating in family education, and providing family therapy. Genograms, or diagrams of family members' relationships, can be a useful tool for the specialist in obtaining information about the family.

KEY WORDS

Couple therapy
Culturally diverse family
Dysfunctional family
Family life cycle

Family therapy
Family therapy stages
Genogram

■ Classroom Teaching Strategies

1. Have students create a genogram of their family going back at least three generations. Have them discuss the uses of the genogram in clinical practice, what they learned about their own family during the exercise, and how they might facilitate a client's completion of his or her own family genogram.

2. Ask students to describe and provide one example for each of the eight phases of family development identified by Duvall (1977). Have students define the stage of family development that their family of origin is currently in. Alternatively, if the class is a more mature group of nontraditional students, have them define and discuss the stage of family development that their own family is in currently.

3. Divide the class in half. One half of the class is charged with the task of creating an argument for why Duvall's family stages are useful as a clinical tool in today's social environment. The other half of the class is charged with the task of creating an argument for why Duvall's family stages are no longer applicable and may be difficult to translate to today's society. Ask each group to provide a rationale and examples for their arguments.

4. Have students discuss culturally diverse families or individuals with whom they have worked in their clinical rotations. If they have not had clinical, ask them to draw from their own personal experiences or their experiences in school. Have students: 1) discuss the cultural issues that influence family behavior in this culture; 2) discuss how the cultural influences might create a situation in which the family could be seen as "not normal" or "dysfunctional" according to middle-class American standards; and 3) talk about ways that nurses can assess and intervene in culturally sensitive ways with a family of this culture.

5. Have students compare and contrast the characteristics of functional and dysfunctional families.

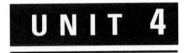

UNIT 4

Special Treatment Modalities

CHAPTER 14

Psychopharmacology

■ Chapter Summary

Psychopharmacology is the study of the mediation and modulation of emotions, behavior, and cognition through the interactions of endogenous signaling substances or chemicals such as dopamine, glutamate, or serotonin and drugs. Changes in emotions, behavior, and cognition result from the use of psychotropic or psychoactive drugs. There are six major classifications of psychotropic agents: 1) antipsychotic agents; 2) hypnotics and antianxiety agents; 3) antidepressants and mood elevators; 4) antimanic agents; 5) anticonvulsants; and 6) anticholinergic or antiparkinson agents. Each of the classes of psychotropic agents has different mechanisms of action, target symptoms, and side effects. This chapter focuses on the different categories of psychotropic agents, rationale for therapy, contraindications, side effects, implications for nursing actions, and client education. Drug polymorphism, or understanding the myriad of factors that can affect the way a drug acts upon the body and mind, has been of increasing interest as clinicians have become more culturally competent in treating psychiatric disorders.

■ Chapter Outline

I. MEDICATING THE PSYCHIATRIC–MENTAL HEALTH CLIENT
    In the past decade, the psychiatric community has become increasingly reliant on psychotropic medications in treating clients. There are clinical guidelines that must be considered when medicating the client who has clinical symptoms of a psychiatric disorder (Burnstein, 1998).

II. THE SCIENCE OF PSYCHOPHARMACOLOGY
    Pharmacokinetics (the movement of drugs and their metabolites through the body) and *pharmacodynamics* (the study of biochemical and physiologic effects of drugs and the ways in which effects are produced) are important terms to know when learning about psychopharmacology. Psychotropic drugs are chemicals that affect the brain and nervous system.

III. ANTIPSYCHOTIC AGENTS

Antipsychotic agents are used clinically to treat most forms of psychosis such as schizophrenia, schizoaffective disorder, affective disorders with psychosis, and psychoses associated with delirium and dementia. Antipsychotic agents that produce neurologic side effects have been called typical antipsychotic drugs, or neuroleptics; their major physiologic action is through dopamine blockade. New-generation antipsychotics (atypical antipsychotics) work by blocking both serotonin and dopamine.

A. Contraindications and Side Effects

There are contraindications that must be considered when prescribing antipsychotics. Side effects may also occur due to the use of antipsychotic medication or due to drug–drug interactions if the client is taking other medications. Common side effects include: drowsiness, inactivity, dry mouth, nasal congestion, blurred vision, skin reactions, pigmentation, photosensitivity, constipation, urinary retention, orthostatic hypotension, diminished libido, seizures, agranulocytosis, ECG changes, gastrointestinal (GI) distress, weight gain, and edema.

The main neuromuscular or neurologic side effects of atypical antipsychotics include extrapyramidal side effects, or EPS (these are acute dyskinesia, parkinsonism, and akathisia); tardive dyskinesia (TD); and neuroleptic malignant syndrome (NMS). EPS is more often an early side effect, while TD may occur after short-term or moderate doses, but more often occurs after long-term use. NMS can occur very suddenly between 1 to 7 days after initiation of therapy or as late as 2 months into therapy.

B. Implications for Nursing Actions

Clients receiving antipsychotic drug therapy should have an evaluation of blood pressure, complete blood count, liver function tests, and vision tests before therapy and at periodic intervals thereafter. There are many guidelines and assessments to consider when caring for the individual who is taking antipsychotic medications, such as give at bedtime, avoid skin contact, mix liquids with fruit juice, do not give subcutaneously, and assess for untoward effects. Psychiatric nurses need to be alert to these, and aware of areas that need frequent observation. Tools such as the Abnormal Involuntary Movement Scale (AIMS) and the Antipsychotic Drug Use Assessment Form are helpful to psychiatric nurses to evaluate medication efficacy and to monitor for side effects.

C. Client Education

Clients need to be informed about the drug therapy, length of time for therapeutic effects to occur, and possible side effects of drug therapy. Instruct clients that psychotropic effects are compounded when given with anxiolytics and sedative-hypnotics; they should avoid sunlight, avoid changing dosage without advice of a physician, avoid antacids, be aware of dizziness, maintain good oral hygiene, and keep pills out of reach of children.

IV. HYPNOTICS AND ANTIANXIETY AGENTS

Hypnotics and antianxiety agents are referred to collectively as hypnosedatives. They are used to treat insomnia, anxiety, tension, alcohol withdrawal, and convulsions and to produce musculoskeletal relaxation. Antianxiety agents can be classified as follows: benzodiazepines, nonbenzodiazepines, antihistamines, beta blockers, hypnotics, and selective serotonin reuptake inhibitors (SSRIs).

A. Benzodiazepines
Benzodiazepines work selectively on the limbic system of the brain, which is responsible for emotions such as rage and anxiety. They produce tranquilizing effects. Side effects can include ataxia and slurred speech. Long-term use of benzodiazepines is not recommended because these drugs are addictive.

B. Nonbenzodiazepines
These are medications that typically block the release of serotonin and prevent the uptake of dopamine. They are less sedating and cause fewer side effects than the benzodiazepines.

C. Antihistamines
Many antihistamines are available to treat a wide variety of medical problems, such as allergies, motion sickness, nausea and vomiting, and drug-induced EPS. Common side effects include drowsiness and dizziness, and they must be used carefully in elderly clients.

D. Beta Blockers
The beta blockers are used to reduce tachycardia, impulsivity, and agitation associated with anxiety. Adverse side effects include hypotension, bradycardia, dizziness, and GI upset, for example.

E. SSRIs and an Atypical Antidepressant
The SSRIs are useful for treating anxiety disorders, although they are categorized as antidepressants.

Implications for Nursing Actions: Before administering hypnotics or antianxiety agents, the nurse should assess the client's mental and physical status to avoid the risk of adverse side effects. The psychiatric nurse needs to be aware of guidelines for nursing interventions during antianxiety or hypnotic drug therapy, including to give at bedtime, give intramuscular doses slowly into large muscles, and frequently assess for adverse effects and drug interactions

Client Education: Clients should be told the name of the drug they are prescribed, the dosage, and the expected course of treatment.

In general, patients should be taught to avoid mixing hypnotics or antianxiety agents with alcoholic beverages, antihistamines, and antipsychotic drugs; to avoid caffeinated beverages; to report side effects; not to stop taking drugs without physician consultation; to avoid long-term use; and that these drugs are not effective as analgesics. In addition, specific guidelines for patient education should be followed for each category of drug.

V. ANTIDEPRESSANTS AND MOOD ELEVATORS

Antidepressants are used to treat depressive disorders. These drugs are classified as tricyclic antidepressants (TCAs), monoamine oxidase inhibitors (MAOIs), SSRIs, and atypical antidepressants. For each classification of drug, the psychiatric nurse must be familiar with the specific contraindications and side effects, implications for nursing actions, and client education for that particular class and type of drug.

A. Tricyclic Antidepressants

The tricyclic antidepressants work by increasing the level of the neurotransmitters serotonin or norepinephrine in the space between the nerve endings.

1. Contraindications and Side Effects: Contraindications include recent myocardial infarction, pregnancy, nursing mothers, and severe liver or kidney disease. Side effects include dry mouth, blurred vision, tachycardia, urinary retention, and constipation.

2. Implications for Nursing Actions: Assess suicidal ideation, side effects, drug interactions, plasma drug levels.

3. Client Education: Avoid over-the-counter drugs, inform dentist and surgeon of drugs taken, report side effects, avoid excessive exercise and high temperatures.

B. Monoamine Oxidase Inhibitors

MAOIs work by preventing the metabolism of neurotransmitters.

1. Contraindications and Side Effects: Contraindications include asthma, cerebral vascular disease, congestive heart failure, hypertension, kidney or liver disease, hypernatremia, cardiac dysrhythmias, pheochromocytoma, hyperthyroidism, severe headaches, alcoholism, glaucoma, colitis, paranoid schizophrenia, debilitation, clients over 60 or under 16, and pregnancy. Side effects are: orthostatic hypotension, drowsiness, insomnia, abnormal heart rate, headache, dizziness, blurred vision, vertigo, constipation, weakness, dry mouth, nausea, vomiting, anorexia, and malignant hypertension with tyramine-rich foods.

2. Implications for Nursing Actions: Tyramine-rich foods taken with MAOIs result in malignant hypertension; Regitine treats hypertensive crisis.

3. Client Education: The patient taking MAOIs must be taught to avoid tyramine-rich foods: aged cheese, avocados, bananas,

chicken livers, fava beans, canned figs, meat tenderizers, pickled herring, raisins, sour cream, soy sauce, yogurt, beer, red wine, and yeast supplements.

C. Selective Serotonin Reuptake Inhibitors
SSRIs work by acting on the reuptake of serotonin in several ways.
1. Contraindications and Side Effects: A period of 14 days is needed for drug clearance if the patient has been taking MAOIs; use caution when client is taking anticoagulants; lower doses of theophylline and alprazolam are necessary; avoid use in clients taking Haldol, Seldane, Valium, alcohol, and tryptophan. Side effects of SSRIs include nausea, diarrhea, constipation, tremor, insomnia, somnolence, dry mouth, headaches, nervousness, anorexia, weight loss, sweating, and sexual dysfunction.
2. Implications for Nursing Actions: Assess suicidal ideation, side effects, drug interactions, plasma drug levels.
3. Client Education: Discuss discontinuing with physician, report unusual symptoms, avoid operating hazardous machinery if drowsiness occurs, and keep out of the reach of children.

D. Mood Elevators
Mood elevators include stimulants such as dextroamphetamine (Dexedrine), methylphenidate (Ritalin), and pemoline (Cylert), for example.

VI. ANTIMANIC AGENTS
Lithium has been considered the treatment of choice for the manic phase of bipolar disorder, although there are three alternate treatment options that are used as well (anticonvulsants, calcium channel antagonists, and atypical antipsychotics). Lithium is thought to produce its effects by augmenting serotonergic function in the central nervous system. It is not metabolized by the body, but 80% is reabsorbed in the kidney and excreted.

A. Contraindications and Side Effects
Contraindications to lithium therapy include pregnancy and impaired kidney function. Common side effects include nausea, metallic taste, abdominal discomfort, polydipsia, polyuria, muscle weakness, fine hand tremors, fatigue, mild diarrhea, and edema. Toxic side effects include drowsiness, slurred speech, muscle spasms, blurred vision, diarrhea, dizziness, stupor, convulsions, coma, and death. Toxicity occurs when serum lithium levels exceed 1.5 to 2.0 mEq/L.

B. Implications for Nursing Actions
Nurses should observe the client carefully for therapeutic effects of lithium, as well as side effects. In addition, nurses should be sure lithium is given with meals, that frequent lithium levels are drawn, that diuretics and anti-inflammatory drugs are avoided, and that

there is adequate sodium and fluid balance.
C. Client Education
Nurses should instruct patients to avoid altering dosage without
physician consultation, monitor salt and fluid balance, avoid fad
diets, avoid excessive exercise, obtain frequent lithium levels,
inform physician of all drugs used, report symptoms, avoid breast
feeding, and maintain regular medical checkups.

VII. ANTICONVULSANTS
Anticonvulsant drugs are used to treat seizure disorders as well as
during alcohol withdrawal and in clients with delirium and dementia
associated with certain physical disorders. There are several classes of
anticonvulsants, including long-acting barbiturates, benzodiazepines,
hydantoins, and succinimides.
A. Contraindications and Side Effects
Contraindications include central nervous system depression,
hepatic or renal damage, bone-marrow depression, pregnancy, and
nursing mothers. Side effects include drowsiness, sedation, ataxia,
GI irritation, skin disorders, blood dyscrasias, respiratory
depression, liver damage, gingival hyperplasia, hypocalcemia, and
lymphadenopathy.
B. Implications for Nursing Actions
Important nursing actions are to give on a round-the-clock schedule
to maintain blood levels, to administer with food, and to observe
for therapeutic and side effects.
C. Client Education
Inform physician about illnesses, pregnancy, and medications taken,
take with food, follow administration directions with Dilantin, and
obtain frequent blood levels.

VIII. ANTIPARKINSON AGENTS
Antiparkinson drugs have been used to treat EPS and include
anticholinergic, antihistaminic, and dopaminergic agents. They block
the action of acetylcholine receptors in the brain and peripheral
nervous system.
A. Contraindications and Side Effects
Contraindications are glaucoma, myasthenia gravis, GI obstruction,
prostatic hypertrophy, and urinary obstruction. Side effects include
orthostatic hypotension, dry mouth, blurred vision, urinary
retention, constipation, and anhidrosis.
B. Implications for Nursing Actions
Give with food and frequently assess therapeutic and side effects.
C. Client Education
Clients need to be taught to maintain adequate fluid intake, avoid

operating hazardous machinery, report side effects, rise slowly to prevent dizziness, avoid strenuous activity in hot weather, get routine medical examinations, and limit intake of alcohol and high-protein foods.

IX. DRUG POLYMORPHISM

Drug polymorphism refers to variation in response to a drug based on a client's age, gender, size, and body composition. In differing ethnic groups, environmental, cultural, and genetic factors can contribute to drug polymorphism.

KEY WORDS

Abnormal Involuntary Movement Scale
Antianxiety agent
Anticonvulsant
Antidepressant
Antihistamines
Antimanic agent
Antiparkinson agent
Atypical antipsychotic
Benzodiazepine
Beta blocker
Discontinuation syndrome
Drug polymorphism
Extrapyramidal effects
Hypertensive crisis
Hypnotic

Lithium
Lithium toxicity
Monoamine oxidase inhibitor
Mood elevator
Neuroleptic malignant syndrome
Nonbenzodiazepine
Pharmacodynamics
Pharmacokinetics
Psychopharmacology
Psychotropic agents
Selective serotonin reuptake inhibitor
Tardive dyskinesia
Tricyclic antidepressants
Typical antipsychotic

■ Classroom Teaching Strategies

1. Assign students the table at the end of the chapter and have them complete the table prior to coming to class. Review and discuss each of the columns during class, providing examples to increase students' understanding of the concepts.

2. Have students discuss nursing interventions and client teaching for each of the psychotropic classes of drugs.

3. Prepare a patient teaching plan for MAOIs, and discuss critical components of client education with these medications.

4. Ask students to think about why patients might be nonadherent with psychotropic medication regimens. Ask for volunteers to discuss the variety of issues that patients must face when dealing with the necessity of controlling symptoms with psychotropic medications.

5. Devise a matching game in which cards with medication names and target symptoms are placed on one side of the board, and psychotropic classification groups are placed on the other. Have students match the appropriate cards to the correct classification groups.

Psychotropic Classification Groups

Drug Class	Examples of Drugs/Dosages in This Class and Target Symptoms	Contra-indications	Side Effects	Nursing Implications	Client Teaching
Antipsychotic Agents					
Hypnotics and Antianxiety Agents					
Antidepressants and Mood Elevators					
Antimanic Agents					
Anticonvulsants					
Anticholinergic or Antiparkinson Agents					

CHAPTER 15

Electroconvulsive Therapy

■ Chapter Summary

The biologic treatment of mental disorders is referred to as somatic therapy. Present-day somatic therapies include clinical psychopharmacology and electroconvulsive therapy (ECT). ECT has proven effective in treating a wide variety of disorders in multiple populations, including children, adolescents, and the elderly. There are relatively few contraindications and side effects of ECT, and it is considered a safe procedure. Nursing interventions focus on teaching the client prior to ECT treatment, preparing the client for treatment, providing care during the procedure, and assisting with posttreatment.

■ Chapter Outline

I. ECT PROCEDURE
Introduced in 1937, ECT uses electric currents to induce convulsive seizures. *Electronarcosis* is a type of ECT that produces a sleep-like state; electrostimulation avoids producing convulsions by using anesthetics and muscle relaxants. ECT delivered to the right side of the brain appears to maximize efficacy while minimizing adverse effects on memory.

II. INDICATIONS FOR USE
ECT is used for clients with depression, schizophrenia, the depressive phase of bipolar disorder, suicidal ideation, therapy-resistant depression, catatonia, pseudodementia, and neuroleptic malignant syndrome. ECT has also been proven effective in treating special populations, such as children, adolescents, and the elderly.

III. CONTRAINDICATIONS TO ECT
Contraindications are assessed in regard to the seriousness and urgency for treatment, and include such conditions as myocardial problems, tuberculosis, recent fractures, hypertension, pregnancy, bleeding or clotting problems, and others.

IV. SIDE EFFECTS

Side effects of ECT include headache, disorientation, and memory disturbance. Also, transient memory loss and impaired cognition often occur. Hyperactive delirium may occur as the client comes out of anesthesia. This may last from a few minutes to an hour, and the client may require intravenous diazepam to stabilize symptoms.

V. ADVANCES IN ECT

The form and dosage of the electrical stimulus and the electrode location contribute to the clinical efficacy and the cognitive effects of seizures. When treatments are not effective, augmentation is considered. This includes changing electrode placement, using an alternate anesthesia, using IV caffeine, and adding other drugs that can augment the effects of ECT.

VI. NURSING INTERVENTIONS

Nursing interventions focus on the following:

A. Teaching the client prior to ECT treatment: Instruction sheets are often given to the client and family, and the procedure is explained in detail. There is a website that provides education and seeks to dispel fears about ECT. It is found at http://www.electroshock.org.

B. Preparing the client for treatment: Focus is on providing a safe environment, monitoring vital signs, alerting team to problems, and providing reassurance to reduce anxiety.

C. Providing care during the procedure: The nurse observes motor seizure in the client, protects extremities, records length of the motor seizure, and monitors the patient closely.

D. Assisting with posttreatment: Recovery interventions are usually conducted by the nurse anesthetist or anesthesiologist until adequate oxygenation, spontaneous respirations, and consciousness and orientation return.

KEY WORDS

Electroconvulsive therapy	Hyperactive delirium
Electronarcosis	Postictal agitation
Electrostimulation	Somatic therapies

■ Classroom Teaching Strategies

1. If possible, during class, use the Internet to look up the website http://www.electroshock.org. Divide the class into groups and have each group survey a portion of the website and report on their findings. Alternatively, have students complete this assignment as a homework exercise, and report on it in class.

2. Ask students to explore their own thoughts and feelings about ECT. Ask for volunteers to share their ideas, and put commonalities on the board. Discuss each issue, and provide evidence or facts to support or refute common beliefs, misconceptions, and/or biases.

3. Show a clip from the movie "One Flew Over the Cuckoo's Nest" in which the character portrayed by Jack Nicholson receives ECT (or, alternatively, assign students to watch this movie for homework). Open the class to discussion about how this movie portrays ECT treatment (is it realistic or not?) and how ECT treatments are done today in reality.

CHAPTER 16

Alternative Therapies

■ Chapter Summary

Alternative therapy, or complementary medicine/therapy, is gaining popularity. Even managed care organizations and insurers are adding such services to their benefits packages. Curing is described as the alleviation of symptoms, while healing is defined as gradual awakening within a person and results in profound change. Holistic nurses use body-mind, spiritual, energetic, and ethical healing. Alternative therapies include such interventions as homeopathic remedies, hypnosis, relaxation therapy, guided imagery, biofeedback, meditation, aromatherapy, acupuncture or acupressure, massage therapy, and therapeutic touch, for example. These therapies are often used to reduce symptoms of pain, insomnia, stress and anxiety, depression, and cognitive decline. The holistic nurse teaches the client self-assessment skills related to emotion, nutrition, activity, sleep–wake cycle, rest, support systems, and spirituality. Clients need education around use of alternative therapies, because adverse side effects and interactions with prescription drugs can cause difficulties if care providers are unaware of the client's use of these therapies.

■ Chapter Outline

I. HOLISTIC NURSING
   Holism is a way of viewing health care in terms of patterns and processes instead of medication, technology, and surgery. Holistic nurses use body-mind, spiritual, energetic, and ethical healing. The American Holistic Nurses' Association has developed standards of care that define the discipline of holistic nursing.

II. USE OF ALTERNATIVE THERAPIES
   Nonpharmaceutical, alternative therapies can be used to relieve a wide variety of clinical symptoms.
   A. Pain
      Several forms of complementary or alternative therapies are used to reduce pain, including homeopathic remedies, hypnosis, relaxation therapy, guided imagery, biofeedback, meditation, aromatherapy,

acupuncture or acupressure, massage therapy, and therapeutic touch.

B. Insomnia
Two natural remedies have been used to treat insomnia: melatonin and valerian. In addition, aromatherapy may also provide sedative or hypnotic effects.

C. Stress and Anxiety
Alternative therapies that have been helpful for stress and anxiety include hypnosis, biofeedback, massage therapy, therapeutic touch, meditation, and aromatherapy. Also, natural remedies such as kava-kava, passionflower, and valerian are used.

D. Depression
Therapeutic touch or massage, acupuncture, aromatherapy, and natural remedies such as St. John's wort and SAM-e are frequently used to minimize symptoms of clinical depression.

E. Cognitive Decline
Gingko biloba is a popular herb that is used to improve blood flow in the brain and to alleviate vertigo and ringing in the ears. It is also used to improve cognition.

III. THE NURSING PROCESS
The holistic nurse teaches the client self-assessment skills related to emotion, nutrition, activity, sleep–wake cycle, rest, support systems, and spirituality. Once the client self-assesses, problems are identified and the client is assisted with problem-solving skills. The client and nurse discuss mutually agreed-upon goals and outcomes. The nurse is a support, coach, and assessor as the client participates in the intervention process. The client is a partner in all aspects of the holistic nursing process.

Clients need education around use of alternative therapies. Adverse side effects and interactions with prescription drugs can cause difficulties if the client is not forthcoming to the health care provider about his or her alternative therapy use. Concern is also raised about the shelf life of some remedies, as well as the lack of standardization of doses. Several Internet websites provide client education.

KEY WORDS

Alternative therapy
Complementary medicine

Holism
Holistic nursing

■ Classroom Teaching Strategies

1. Ask students to find recent newspaper clippings or website articles about alternative therapies and natural remedies. Have them bring these to class, and use as a point for discussion about the current popularity and pitfalls of such therapies.

2. Divide the class into groups, and assign each group to one of the following symptoms: pain, insomnia, cognitive decline, stress and anxiety, and depression.

   Instruct each group to prepare a brief presentation for the class on the types of alternative therapies that are commonly used for each symptom category. Have them discuss pros and cons of such use.

3. Ask students to consider a time when they may have considered using alternative therapies. Discuss the reasons why they considered this, and why or why not they might encourage clients to do so.

4. Have students role–play being a nurse in a primary care office. How would they, as the nurse, ask the client about the use of alternative therapies? What are ways that would encourage the client to be open about this; are there ways that might discourage the sharing of this information?

5. Ask students to discuss reasons why clients might not be safe in using alternative therapies, providing examples.

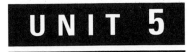
UNIT 5

Clients
With Psychiatric
Disorders

CHAPTER 17

Schizophrenia and Other Psychotic Disorders

■ Chapter Summary

Schizophrenia is the most common and disabling of the psychiatric disorders. This chapter focuses on the causes and types of schizophrenia, symptoms exhibited, treatments, and nursing interventions. Etiologic theories include genetic, biochemical and neurostructural, organic or psychophysiologic, environment/culture, perinatal, psychological/experiential, and vitamin deficiency theories. Symptoms are diverse and include positive symptoms (such as hallucinations and delusions), negative symptoms (such as withdrawal), and disorganized symptoms (such as incoherent or disorganized speech). There are five subtypes of schizophrenia: paranoid, catatonic, disorganized, undifferentiated, and residual. In addition, there are five subtypes of schizophrenic-like disorders: schizoaffective disorder; schizophreniform disorder; brief psychotic disorder; psychotic disorder; and shared psychotic disorder. Cultural considerations are important when diagnosing, assessing symptoms, and managing care. The nursing process is addressed, including strategies for assessment, nursing diagnosis, outcome identification, interventions, implementation, and evaluation. Client and family education is critical, and the continuum of care must be addressed to reduce recidivism.

■ Chapter Outline

I. CAUSES
   A. Genetic Theory
      The genetic, or hereditary, predisposition theory holds that there are genetic links to schizophrenia—possibly chromosome deletion syndrome, genetic links found to chromosomes 13 and 8. Studies continue on genome scanning and DNA marker technology.
   B. Biochemical and Neurostructural Theory
      Dopamine Hypothesis: Excessive dopamine bombards brain nerve impulses. Also abnormalities of brain shape and circuitry are being studied.

C. Organic or Psychophysiologic Theory
Perhaps a functional deficit; caused by stressors (viral infections, toxins, trauma, abnormal substances) or metabolic disorder.

D. Environmental or Cultural Theory
Faulty reaction to environment; person is unable to respond selectively to numerous social stimuli.

E. Perinatal Theory
Fetus or newborn is deprived of oxygen or mother suffers from malnutrition during first trimester.

F. Psychological or Experiential Theory
Prefrontal lobes are responsive to environmental stress; stressors may contribute to onset, including poor mother–child relationships; disturbed family relationships; impaired sexual identity/body image; repeated exposure to double-bind communication.

G. Vitamin Deficiency Theory
Possible deficiencies in vitamin B, especially B_1, B_6, and B_{12}; and vitamin C.

II. CLINICAL SYMPTOMS
May appear suddenly or develop over time. Bleuler (1857–1939) introduced term "schizophrenia" and classified symptoms into "four A's": affective disturbance, autistic thinking, ambivalence, and looseness of associations. Symptoms fall into three categories: positive symptoms (presence of psychotic or distorted behavior), negative symptoms (diminution or loss of normal functions), and disorganized symptoms (confused thinking, disorganization). Type I: Positive symptoms have acute onset and respond to neuroleptic medications. Type II: Negative symptoms have slow onset; respond best to atypical antipsychotics.

III. DIAGNOSTIC CRITERIA

A. Paranoid Type
Persecutory delusions; hallucinations; behavior changes.

B. Catatonic Type
Psychomotor disturbance; delusions during withdrawn state.

C. Disorganized Type
Most severe of all subtypes. Disintegration of personality; withdrawal; incoherent speech; uninhibited behavior. Prognosis is poor.

D. Undifferentiated Type
Atypical symptoms that do not meet criteria for other subtypes.

E. Residual Type
The experience of negative symptoms following at least one acute episode.

IV. SCHIZOPHRENIC-LIKE DISORDERS

Five subtypes: schizoaffective disorder (uninterrupted period of illness with major depressive, manic, or mixed episode plus negative symptoms); schizophreniform disorder (features of schizophrenia for more than 1 but less than 6 months); brief psychotic disorder (sudden onset; at least one positive symptom); psychotic disorder (prominent hallucinations or delusions due to medical condition); and shared psychotic disorder (two people who share the same delusion; see Chapter 18).

V. TRANSCULTURAL CONSIDERATIONS

Consider cultural differences when assessing symptoms. Culture may play a role in the expression of various symptoms that may be acceptable in one culture and not in another. There is a tendency to overdiagnose schizophrenia in some ethnic groups.

VI. THE NURSING PROCESS

A. Assessment

Communication; subjective data from family members; side effects of medications; support systems; activities of daily living; bizarre eating habits. Document physical conditions, congruence of mood with affect. Assess psychogenic polydipsia (compulsive behavior of drinking 3 or more liters of fluid per day).

B. Nursing Diagnoses

Consider acute versus chronic symptom onset; decompensation; case management needs.

C. Outcome Identification

Influenced by severity of disorder; support system availability; clinical setting of treatment.

D. Planning Interventions

Consider biological, cognitive, perceptual, behavioral, and emotional disturbances. Medication may be required; cognitive, behavioral, and other supportive therapies. Integrated approach to interventions; addressing continuum of care, community treatment programs, vocational rehabilitation beneficial.

E. Implementation

Focus on establishing trust; open communication; safe environment; alleviation of symptoms; maintaining biologic integrity. Interventions include encouragement; simple communications; structured environment; protection from self-harm; limit setting; time out; physical restraints; medication and side effect management. Earlier treatment leads to better outcomes.

F. Evaluation

Purpose is to compare current mental status with stated outcome criteria.

KEY WORDS

Awareness syndrome

Bleuler's four A's

Catatonic

Disorganized symptoms

Dopamine hypothesis

Negative symptoms

Paranoid

Positive symptoms

Psychogenic polydipsia

Schizoaffective disorde

Schizophreniform disorder

■ Classroom Teaching Strategies

1. Ask students to use the Internet to explore cases of schizophrenia or schizophrenia-like disorders of individuals in the news (e.g., Mark Chapman) or, alternatively, to seek out movies that portray schizophrenia-like symptoms (e.g., "One Flew Over the Cuckoo's Nest" or "The Shining"). Have students discuss the symptoms that are reported and the way in which the disorder is portrayed, and whether or not the reports are reality-based or erroneous overdramatizations. If possible, encourage students to bring in film clips that demonstrate particular symptoms. Ask students to report in class on their findings and discussion.

2. Engage students in a discussion of what they believe the most difficult symptoms or behaviors would be to manage with the schizophrenic disorders. Discuss why the behavior would be difficult, and what the nurse might do to overcome his or her own feelings and thoughts and to intervene with the behavior.

3. Ask students to develop a plan of care for educating the spouse of a newly diagnosed person with schizophrenia. What areas would the nurse need to focus on, and why? What would be the critically important facts for educating the family?

4. Present a case study of a 19-year-old college student with acute-onset schizophrenia. Divide the class into groups to discuss and present: 1) symptoms and associated behaviors that merit the diagnosis; 2) social and cultural issues that may be salient; 3) suggested interventions for problematic behaviors; and 4) their own thoughts and feelings that might emerge if they were assigned to care for this individual.

5. Ask students to discuss Bleuler's four A's and how they have been translated into today's diagnostic criteria. Discuss symptoms and behaviors and treatments that are more and less effective for each symptom. Discuss how the care of individuals with schizophrenia has changed since the early 1900s.

CHAPTER 18

Delusional Disorders

■ Chapter Summary

Delusional disorders are characterized by delusional thought. These disorders can result from a variety of causes, such as relocation, sensory handicaps, severe stress, low socioeconomic status, trust–fear conflicts, and identifiable neurologic disease. There are several types of delusional disorders: dementia, substance-induced psychotic disorder, schizophrenia, psychotic disorder due to a medical condition, mood disorder, paranoid personality disorder, delusional disorder, and shared psychotic disorder. Five subtypes of delusional disorder, each with unique symptoms and behaviors, include persecutory, conjugal, erotomanic, grandiose, and somatic. The nursing process for the delusional client includes assessment, diagnosis, outcome identification, intervention, implementation, and evaluation. Treating the delusional client is most often done on an outpatient basis and includes interventions that foster the therapeutic relationship; decreasing fear and suspicion, hostility, aggression, and delusions; observing for suicidal ideation; and assisting the client with activities of daily living. Cultural and social issues must be taken into consideration when assessing and treating delusional individuals.

■ Chapter Outline

I. CAUSES
   Predisposing factors identified include: relocation; sensory handicaps; severe stress; low socioeconomic status; trust–fear conflicts. Delusions can result from identifiable neurologic diseases (these are called content-specific delusions, or CDCs), associated with generalized or systemic disorders, such as hypothyroid disease.

II. CLINICAL SYMPTOMS
   Age of onset usually middle or late adult life. Symptoms include delusions of suspiciousness and distrust, paranoia; complaints about injustices; social isolation, seclusiveness, or eccentric behavior; anxiety or depression.

III. DIAGNOSTIC CRITERIA
Delusional disorders are characterized by delusional thought. Several types: dementia; substance-induced psychotic disorder; psychotic disorder due to medical condition; mood disorder; paranoid personality disorder; delusional disorder; and shared psychotic disorder.
  A. Delusional Disorder
  Different from schizophrenia in that audiovisual hallucinations do not usually occur and delusions are not bizarre. Clients refuse to acknowledge negative feelings, thoughts, motives, or behaviors in themselves, and can have ideas of reference (self-centered thoughts in which everything is taken personally).
    1. Five Subtypes of Delusional Disorder
      a. Persecutory: belief that one is being conspired against, spied on, poisoned, or obstructed in some way.
      b. Conjugal or jealous: belief that mate is unfaithful
      c. Erotomanic: belief that a person of elevated status loves one
      d. Grandiose: belief that one possesses unrecognized talent or insight and seeks position of power.
      e. Somatic: preoccupation with body and somatic complaints
  B. Shared Psychotic Disorder
  Also called "folie à deux": two people with close relationship who share same delusion. Often related, have lived together for a long time, and may be socially isolated.

IV. TRANSCULTURAL CONSIDERATIONS
Delusional content varies from culture to culture and reflects cultural patterns. Important to assess cultural context of delusions.

V. THE NURSING PROCESS
  A. Assessment
  Challenging because person often denies pathology and is suspicious, untrusting, and resistive to therapy. Include cultural and religious background; behavioral disturbances; depression; anxiety; economic stability; self-esteem; impaired social, occupational, or marital functioning.
  B. Nursing Diagnoses
  May include disturbed thought processes; impaired social interaction.
  C. Outcome Identification
  Depends on severity of disorder and ability of client for self-care in community. Focus on identifying situations that evoke symptoms; minimizing delusions; identifying problems with relationships; stabilizing relationships; differentiating between fantasy and reality.

D. Planning Interventions
   May occur in private practice or mental health clinic. Nurse should demonstrate self-awareness of own thoughts and feelings about caring for delusional clients.

E. Implementation
   Focus on establishing rapport; enhancing self-esteem; decreasing suspicion, hostility, aggression, and delusions; observe for suicidal ideation; and assist with ADL. Insight-oriented, problem-solving, and group therapies may be ineffective.

F. Evaluation
   Purpose is to compare current mental status with desirable outcome criteria.

KEY WORDS

Conjugal delusions
Content-specific delusions
Delusional
Erotomania
Folie à deux

Grandiosity
Ideas of reference
Paranoid
Persecutory delusions

■ Classroom Teaching Strategies

1. Divide the class into five groups. Distribute five index cards (one for each group) on which are written one of the five nonproductive reactions to delusional clients identified by Barile (1984): 1) becoming anxious and avoiding the client; 2) reinforcing delusions by actually believing the client; 3) attempting to prove that the client is mistaken by presenting a logical argument; 4) setting unrealistic goals that lead to disappointment, frustration, or anger; and 5) being inconsistent with nursing interventions. Ask students to 1) demonstrate the nonproductive reaction in a clinical vignette and 2) replay the vignette and replace the nonproductive reaction with a productive, therapeutic one. Discuss what is nonproductive or therapeutic about each intervention.

2. Use clips from a relevant movie (for example, "Conspiracy Theory" or "One Flew Over the Cuckoo's Nest") to illustrate symptoms of a delusional disorder. Discuss whether or not symptoms are portrayed accurately and treated appropriately, and how the individual with symptoms is treated. Use as a point for discussing the media's portrayal of mental illness.

3. Assign students the task of searching for cultures that may engage in behaviors or rituals that could be considered delusional in modern-day American culture. Examples might include cultures in which voodoo is

practiced, or religious or spiritual rites that are unusual. Have them bring their findings to the class and report on them.

4. Ask students to write down one delusional behavior that they feel would be the most difficult for them to handle, and why. Explore common reactions and feelings to delusional behaviors and thoughts; include the nursing role in self-exploration and techniques to handle and intervene with one's own countertransference.

5. Present a brief case study of a delusional client, including specific symptoms, severity, duration, social supports, activities of daily living, and occupational functioning. Discuss areas for further assessment, planning, and intervention. Assist students to highlight areas of importance in assessing the delusional client and addressing functional deficits with appropriate nursing interventions.

CHAPTER 19

Mood Disorders

■ Chapter Summary

Depression is one of the most common psychiatric disorders by any measure, and it can occur at any age. About 50% of depression cases are underdiagnosed and undertreated by nonpsychiatric practitioners. This chapter focuses on the causes of depression, including genetic and biologic predisposition; biochemical; psychodynamic; behavioral; cognitive; and environmental theories. Risk factors and clinical symptoms are also addressed. Types of depressive disorders are outlined, such as major depressive disorder; dysthymic; cyclothymic; and bipolar I and II disorders. Components of the nursing process are reviewed: assessment, nursing diagnoses, outcome identification, planning interventions, implementation, and evaluation.

■ Chapter Outline

I. CAUSES OF DEPRESSION
  A. Genetic and Biologic Predisposition Theory
     A dominant gene may influence or predispose a person to react more to loss or grief, thus becoming depressed. It may be that reduced blood flow and glucose metabolism are culprits, and studies have found a relationship between cerebral biochemistry and symptom severity.
  B. Biochemical Theory
     The biogenic amine hypothesis holds that biogenic amines (norepinephrine and serotonin) at brain receptor sites may be reduced, causing depression. Elevated cortisol levels are also found in depression, as are low thyroid hormone levels.
  C. Psychodynamic Theory
     This theory begins with the observation that bereavement normally produces symptoms resembling depression. After the loss of an important loved person, any loss or disappointment in later life reactivates delayed grief, accompanied by self-criticism, guilt, and anger turned inward.

91

D. Behavioral Theory: Learned Helplessness
Behaviorists regard depression as a form of acquired or learned behavior. The individual has a perception that things are beyond his or her control and thus feels hopeless and helpless, both hallmarks of depression.

E. Cognitive Theory
This theory holds that thoughts are maintained by reinforcement and contribute to depression. Self-defeating thoughts become part of a destructive cycle in which the individual is apathetic, sad, and socially withdrawn.

F. Environmental Theory
Environmental stresses can contribute to depression, including dramatic changes in one's life, financial hardship, physical illness, perceived or real failure, and midlife crises, for example.

II. RISK FACTORS FOR DEPRESSION
Risk factors include prior episodes and family history of depression, prior suicide attempts, female gender, age of onset less than 40 years, postpartum period, medical comorbidity, lack of social support, stressful life events, alcohol or substance abuse, and presence of other psychiatric conditions.

III. CLINICAL SYMPTOMS OF DEPRESSION
Depression has been classified many ways; one is on a continuum from mild to severe depression. Mild depression is transient. Moderate depression (dysthymia) is less severe than major depressive disorder. Severe depression causes psychotic symptoms. Major depressive disorders (endogenous depression) occur when the depression develops from within and there is no apparent cause.

IV. DIAGNOSTIC CRITERIA FOR DEPRESSIVE DISORDERS
A. Major Depressive Disorder
Person does not exhibit momentary shifts of mood and has at least five symptoms that interfere with functioning.

B. Dysthymic Disorder
Not as severe as major depressive disorder, and person does not have delusions, hallucinations, impaired communication, or incoherence. Is usually persistent for 2 years or more.

C. Depressive Disorder Not Otherwise Specified
Used to identify disorders with depressive features that do not meet other criteria for depressive illnesses.

V. DIAGNOSTIC CRITERIA FOR BIPOLAR DISORDERS
A. Bipolar I Disorder
A recurrent disorder in which the person has one or more manic episodes or mixed episodes. When manic, the person has elevated,

expansive, or irritable mood lasting at least 1 week, and there is significant functional impairment.

B. Bipolar II Disorder
Characterized by recurrent major depressive episodes, with hypomanic (a mood between euphoria and excessive elation) episodes. More frequent in women than men.

C. Cyclothymic Disorder
Numerous periods of hypomanic symptoms and depressive symptoms that do not meet criteria for a major depressive episode. Symptoms occur for at least 2 years, and do not subside for more than 2 months at a time.

VI. OTHER MOOD DISORDERS

A. Mood Disorder Due to a General Medical Condition
Some medications and general medical conditions are associated with an increased risk of depression. Client exhibits prominent and persistent mood disturbance that is depressed, elevated, expansive, or irritable, and has significant functional impairment.

VII. TRANSCULTURAL CONSIDERATIONS
Cultures may differ in terms of depressive symptoms and in their judgments about the seriousness of clinical symptoms.

VIII. THE NURSING PROCESS

A. Assessment
Assessment is sometimes difficult with depressed clients and focuses on mood, affect, behavior, cognition, appearance, sleep patterns, attention span, concentration, appetite, and suicidal thoughts. Risk factors should be assessed. Information is important regarding prior treatment, antidepressant medication, and alternative therapies. Input by family and significant others is also important.

B. Nursing Diagnoses
Factors influencing formulation of nursing diagnoses include medical condition, activities of daily living, level of depression, and suicidal ideation or plan.

C. Outcome Identification
Focuses on safety and security, physical health, acceptance and belonging, positive self-concept, and empowerment. For manic clients, also channeling energy and perceiving reality accurately are important to assess.

D. Planning Interventions
Most mood disorders are time-limited and respond well to medication. Nurse must also be aware of personal predisposition to depression and to his or her moods and feelings when treating these

clients. In caring for the client, nurses should display acceptance, honesty, empathy, and patience. Safety is a critical issue, and frequent assessments, for suicidal and self-destructive impulses are key.

E. Implementation
  1. Assistance in Meeting Basic Needs: Nurse assists client in meeting basic needs by assisting with bathing, grooming, personal hygiene, attire, diet, intake and output, rest and activity, and limit setting, when appropriate.
  2. Medication Management: Monitoring medication compliance and side effects is critical. Most antidepressant medication takes 2 to 3 weeks to take effect. Clients may stop taking medications when they begin to feel better.
  3. Somatic Therapies: Electroconvulsive therapy (ECT) and phototherapy have been used. Vagus nerve stimulation (VNS), a newer treatment, is thought to regulate the release of neurotransmitters and can be effective.
  4. Interactive Therapies: Interpersonal, family, group, cognitive, and behavioral psychotherapies, as well as occupational and recreational therapies, have all been shown to be effective in reducing depressive symptoms.
  5. Alternative Therapies: Acupuncture provides significant symptom relief and is under investigation.
  6. Client Education: Focuses on recognizing the onset or recurrence of clinical symptoms of depression or mania; understanding dynamics; recognizing side effects; and establishing a support system.

F. Evaluation
  Response to interventions is evaluated in an ongoing way based on the attainment of desired outcomes.

KEY WORDS

Biogenic amine theory	Hypomania
Bipolar I and II disorder	Learned helplessness
Cyclothymic disorder	Mania
Dysthymia	Phototherapy
ECT	Somatic therapies

■ Classroom Teaching Strategies

1. Provide the following vignette for students, and give them time to formulate their plan during class and to present their findings:
   "You are assigned to take care of Ms. J, a woman who is admitted for

major depressive disorder. She is verbalizing suicidal ideas. Formulate your areas for comprehensive assessment, diagnosis, and nursing intervention to care for Ms. J., emphasizing safety as the number one priority."

2. Use the following vignette to stimulate a discussion of cultural issues with depression:

   "You are working with a young Haitian client, Ms. Q, who has recently moved to the United States from Haiti. You enter her bedroom and find her chanting with words that are unfamiliar to you, and holding a small doll. Discuss what you might be thinking and feeling, how you might assess Ms. Q further, and what types of interventions would be appropriate and not appropriate."

3. Ask patients to compare and contrast symptoms of major depression and mania, including interventions that would be appropriate for one and not for the other.

4. Discuss the nursing care for a client who is started on antidepressant medications during an inpatient stay. Include target symptoms, mechanisms of action, side effects to watch for, and education needed. Discuss how the risk for suicide changes over time with the initiation of psychotropic antidepressants.

5. Write the words *bipolar I, bipolar II,* and *cyclothymic* on the chalkboard. Ask students to come to the board and brainstorm about the differences between these three types of mood disorders and how nursing intervention may differ (or not) between them.

CHAPTER 20

Anxiety Disorders

■ Chapter Summary

Anxiety was first recognized as a medical problem in the 1800s, and Freud introduced anxiety as a psychological concept in the early 1900s. The term "anxiety" describes feelings of uneasiness or tension that a person experiences in response to an unknown object or situation. The term "fear" differs from anxiety in that it is the body's response to a known or recognized danger. There are several terms to describe anxiety, including signal anxiety (response to anticipated event), anxiety trait (personality component), anxiety state (resulting from a stressful situation), and free-floating anxiety (is always present and accompanied by feeling of dread). There are several types of anxiety, and many theories about etiology. Anxiety may be described in terms of phases (normal, acute, chronic, or panic) and levels (euphoria, mild, moderate, severe, and panic state). There are many symptoms of anxiety, including physiologic; psychological or emotional; behavioral; and intellectual or cognitive. This chapter focuses on the theories, clinical symptoms, and nursing process related to the spectrum of anxiety disorders.

■ Chapter Outline

I. CAUSES
   A. Psychoanalytic Theory
      Holds that anxiety results from unresolved, unconscious conflicts between impulses for aggression and the ego's recognition of damage that could result. Newer psychodynamic theories focus on anxiety as an interaction between temperament and environmental factors.
   B. Cognitive Behavioral Theory
      Beck developed the cognitive behavioral theory, suggesting that anxiety is a learned or conditioned response to a stressful event or perceived danger.
   C. Biologic Theory
      Links have been found between anxiety and catecholamines; neuroendocrine measures; neurotransmitters such as serotonin, GABA, and cholecystokinin; and autonomic reactivity.

D. Genetic Theory
One's vulnerability to anxiety disorders may be partially determined by genetics. Studies have suggested that there are some important genes that contribute to the clinical manifestation of anxiety.

E. Social-Cultural Theory
Holds that social or cultural factors cause anxiety, and as the personality develops, the self-concept may be negative, causing difficulty in adapting to everyday demands.

II. CLINICAL SYMPTOMS

There are numerous clinical symptoms, including physiologic, psychological or emotional, and intellectual or cognitive. These may vary according to the level of anxiety being experienced:

A. Levels
1. Level Zero—euphoria: exaggerated feeling of well-being.
2. Level One—mild: increased alertness to inner feelings or the environment.
3. Level Two—moderate: narrowing of the ability to perceive others; focus on only one specific thing.
4. Level Three—severe: focus on small, scattered details; physiologic responses occur at this time.
5. Level Four—panic: complete disruption of ability to perceive; disintegration of personality.

III. DIAGNOSTIC CRITERIA

A. Panic Disorder With or Without Agoraphobia
Characterized by panic attacks that occur "out of the blue"; sudden fright; symptoms may include terror, sense of reality, sense of losing control. Last between a minute and an hour. Symptoms develop suddenly and quickly increase in intensity.

B. Phobic Disorders
1. Agoraphobia
The most common phobic disorder. Fear of being alone in public places.
2. Social Phobia
A compelling desire to avoid situations in which a person may be criticized by others.
3. Specific Phobia
Excessive fear of an object, an activity, or a situation that leads a person to avoid the cause of that fear. Content varies according to culture and ethnicity.

C. Generalized Anxiety Disorders
Commonly seen in primary care settings. Characterized by excessive anxiety and worrying and the following symptoms:

restlessness; fatigue; impaired concentration; irritability; muscle tension; and sleep disturbance.

D. Obsessive–Compulsive Disorder
Characterized by two main symptoms: 1) obsessions: persistent, painful, intrusive thoughts, emotions, or urges that one cannot suppress or ignore; and 2) compulsions: performance of a repetitious, uncontrollable, but seemingly purposeful act to prevent some future event or situations. Ideational compulsion is an urge to carry out an act within one's mind.

E. Post-Traumatic Stress Disorder
Response to trauma such as sexual and other violence, traumatic losses, and war-related trauma. Clinical symptoms include isolation, unpredictable rage, avoidance of feelings, survival guilt, sleep disturbance, nightmares, intrusive thoughts, and depression or anxiety.

F. Acute Stress Disorder
Symptoms occur during or immediately after the trauma, last for at least 2 days, and resolve within 4 weeks after the conclusion of the event. Symptoms include dissociation, such as numbness or detachment; reduced awareness of surroundings; derealization; depersonalization; or dissociative amnesia.

G. Anxiety Disorder Due to a Medical Condition (symptoms are directly related to medical condition; see Chapter 21)

H. Substance-Induced Anxiety Disorder (directly related to abuse of a substance; see Chapter 25)

I. Atypical Anxiety Disorder
A catch-all category for clients exhibiting symptoms that do not meet criteria for any other anxiety disorder.

IV. TRANSCULTURAL CONSIDERATIONS
There is cultural variation in the expression of anxiety. Must consider cultural context, norms, and environmental setting when evaluating symptoms.

V. THE NURSING PROCESS

A. Assessment
First, identify client's level of anxiety. Obtain thorough history, focusing on client's physiologic, emotional, behavioral, and cognitive functioning. Inquire about presence of anxiety; past occurrences with precipitants; frequency and duration of symptoms; and how client coped.

B. Nursing Diagnoses
Challenging because subjective data may be influenced by level of anxiety. Consider activity level, communication, sleep pattern, self-

perception, relationship with others, sexuality, coping skills.

C. Outcome Identification
Consider client's physical status, activity tolerance, severity of symptoms, support systems, and clinical setting for treatment.

D. Planning Interventions
Based on symptom severity, presence of comorbid (medical) conditions, and motivation for treatment.

E. Implementation
Use calm, nonjudgmental approach; short, simple sentences; and firmness; channel client's behavior into outlets for anxiety; anxiolytics may be helpful.

1. Client Education
Can educate one-to-one or in classes or support groups, including family when possible.

2. Techniques to Reduce Anxiety
Techniques that have been effective include: visual imagery; change of pace or scenery; exercise or massage; Transcendental Meditation; biofeedback; systematic desensitization; relaxation exercises; Therapeutic Touch or Healing Touch; hypnosis; and implosion therapy (flooding).

3. Interactive Therapies
Individual psychotherapy, educational and supportive counseling; cognitive behavioral therapy.

4. Other Therapies
Can include exposure therapy, virtual reality, group therapy, family therapy, environmental modification, and alternative therapies.

5. Medication Management
Psychotropic drugs usually reserved for moderate to severe anxiety. Classes used include benzodiazepines, nonbenzodiazepine anxiolytics, antidepressants, beta blockers, and neuroleptics.

F. Evaluation
Focuses on client's response to treatment, understanding of medication management, maintaining social supports.

KEY WORDS

Agoraphobia
Anxiety
Anxiety state
Anxiety trait
Biofeedback
Cognitive behavioral therapy
Compulsion

Implosion therapy
Levels of anxiety
Obsession
Panic disorder
Phases of anxiety
Phobias
Post-traumatic stress disorder

Euphoria	Signal anxiety
Fear	Social phobia
Free-floating anxiety	Systematic desensitization
Healing Touch	Therapeutic Touch
Hypnosis	Transcendental Meditation
Ideational compulsion	

■ Classroom Teaching Strategies

1. Ask the student to make an "anxiety map" of the five levels of anxiety (euphoria, mild, moderate, severe, and panic state) and track a client's move through the levels. Provide a case situation (for example, a client is preparing for a surgical procedure the following day, or a client is facing getting an injection when he or she is needle-phobic). For each level, identify: symptoms that the nurse might observe; the client's responses to his or her anxiety; and specific nursing interventions that would help the client move down a level and interventions that might force the client to move up a level (which would not be therapeutic).

2. Ask students to discuss various techniques that might be useful for anxiety, such as Therapeutic Touch, hypnosis, implosion therapy, systematic desensitization, and so forth. Engage them in a discussion of what might be beneficial for them personally, and why.

3. During class, ask students to massage the shoulders of the person in front of them. After a 5-minute session, ask students to write down the physiologic, psychological or emotional, behavioral, and intellectual or cognitive symptoms they experienced.

4. If possible, obtain a copy of the Spielberger State-Trait Anxiety Scale, and have students complete the scale. Discuss their characteristics, and use this as a tool to discuss assessment of their patient's state and trait anxiety.

5. Present the following case study: "Mr. R. has been admitted to the acute care psychiatric unit with Post-Traumatic Stress Disorder. He is a fireman, and was going into the World Trade Center when it collapsed. He narrowly avoided death; however, he lost six of his best friends in the disaster. Since then (4 months ago), he has experienced recurring flashbacks, nightmares, and suicidal ideation." Discuss appropriate nursing interventions, including the type and level of Mr. R's anxiety and symptoms. What are your priorities for care during the first 24 hours of admission?

CHAPTER 21

Anxiety-Related Disorders

■ Chapter Summary

This chapter presents information about theories of anxiety-related disorders, including Selye's general adaptation syndrome, emotional specificity theory, organ specificity theory, familial theory, and learning theory. Clinical symptoms of various somatoform and dissociative disorders are presented, including features that distinguish them from one another. The nursing process is presented, with assessment, diagnosis, outcome identification, planning interventions, implementation, and evaluation strategies. Addressing medical and cultural issues is important when assessing and intervening with clients who have anxiety-related disorders.

■ Chapter Outline

I. CAUSES
   A. Selye's General Adaptation Syndrome
      When coping with stress, the individual experiences a "fight or flight" response in three stages: alarm reaction, resistance, and exhaustion.
   B. Emotional Specificity Theory
      Specific emotions (such as "type A" personality, which is characterized by impatience, aggressiveness, sense of urgency) have specific effects on physiologic function (such as those with type A personalities are susceptible to coronary artery disease).
   C. Organ Specificity Theory
      The individual responds to stress with a particular organ or system.
   D. Familial Theory
      Dynamic family relationships influence the development of medical disorders. "Psychosomatogenic" family as individuals who develop physiologic symptoms rather than face or resolve conflict.
   E. Learning Theory
      Person learns to produce a physiologic response to achieve reward, attention, or reinforcement, and cannot give up the disorder easily.

II. DIAGNOSTIC CRITERIA

A. Anxiety Disorder Due to a General Medical Condition
Prominent anxiety, panic attacks, or obsessions or compulsions that are due to direct physiologic effects of a medical condition.

B. Psychological Factors (Anxiety) Affecting Medical Condition
Presence of specific psychological or behavioral factors that adversely affect a general medical condition; any medical condition caused or influenced by psychological factors.

C. Somatoform Disorders
Differ from psychological factors affecting medical condition in that somatoform disorders are reflected in disordered physiologic complaints or symptoms, not under voluntary control; clients do not demonstrate organic findings.

1. Body Dysmorphic Disorder
   Preoccupation with an imagined defect in appearance.

2. Somatization Disorder
   Free-floating anxiety disorder; client expresses emotional turmoil or conflict through a physical system.

3. Conversion Disorder
   Psychological condition in which anxiety-provoking impulse is converted unconsciously into functional symptoms. "La belle indifference" refers to the individual's reaction of indifference to symptoms and displaying no anxiety. Different from malingering, which is a conscious effort to feign the symptoms of illness to avoid unpleasant situation or for selfish gain.

4. Pain Disorder
   a. Pain disorder associated with psychological factors: psychological factors have major role in onset, severity, exacerbation, or maintenance of pain.
   b. Pain disorder associated with both psychological factors and general medical condition: pain is predominant focus of clinical presentation; warrants clinical attention.

5. Hypochondriasis
   Unrealistic or exaggerated physical complaints; preoccupied with fear of having disease.

6. Undifferentiated Somatoform Disorder
   One or more physical complaints lasting 6 months or longer; cannot be explained by a known medical condition or from a substance.

7. Somatoform Disorder Not Otherwise Specified
   Used when symptoms do not meet criteria for any specific somatoform disorder.

D. Dissociative Disorders
Essential feature: disruption of integrated functions of consciousness, memory, identity, or perception of the environment.

1. Dissociative Amnesia
   Characterized by inability to recall personal information because of physical or psychological trauma. Amnesia can be circumscribed; selective; generalized; continuous. Clinical features: perplexity, disorientation, purposeless wandering.
2. Dissociative Fugue
   Sudden and unexpected departure from home or work; inability to recall past. Rare occurrence.
3. Dissociative Identity Disorder
   Formerly called multiple personality disorder; person dominated by at least one of two or more definitive personalities at one time.
4. Depersonalization Disorder
   Strange alteration in perception or experience of self; often associated with sense of unreality. Can also have dizziness, depression, anxiety, fear of "going insane," disturbance in subjective sense of time.

III. THE NURSING PROCESS
   A. Assessment
      Thorough biopsychosocial and cultural history; validate data obtained from client. Assess onset of symptoms, psychophysiologic reactions, amount of stress; thorough physical examination.

   B. Nursing Diagnoses
      Diagnoses vary depending on real or perceived comorbid condition or a dissociative disorder.

   C. Outcome Identification
      Focus on client's ability to recognize anxiety, identify stressors, ways to modify or eliminate stressors, develop effective coping skills.

   D. Planning Interventions
      Use holistic, individualized approach. Immediate medical attention may be needed; laboratory tests and x-rays to rule out organicity. Help client develop effective coping skills; identify supportive therapies to reduce anxiety.

   E. Implementation
      Therapeutic relationship is key. Assist with ADL, give detailed explanations about medications, treatments; tell family results of negative physical examination; limit setting; provide structure; reality orientation.
      1. Holistic Approach: identify stressors to reduce their effect or eliminate them. Provide comprehensive treatment.
      2. Project SMART: Stress resistance project, found ways people coped well over 12-year period: including using mastery skills; committing to meaningful project; making wise choices; seeking social support; maintaining humor; concern for others.

F. Evaluation

Review client role, anxiety-producing stressors. Discuss post-treatment continuum of care and follow-up.

KEY WORDS

Body dysmorphic disorder

Conversion disorder

Depersonalization

Dissociative amnesia

Dissociative identity disorder

General adaptation syndrome

Hypochondriasis

La belle indifference

Malingering

Organ specificity theory

Primary gain

Project SMART

Secondary gain

Somatization

Somatoform disorder

Type A personality

■ Classroom Teaching Strategies

1. Divide class into three sections, and assign each section one stage of Selye's general adaptation syndrome (alarm reaction, resistance, and exhaustion). Have each group provide a clinical vignette illustrating symptoms of the stage and physiologic responses in each stage. Identify nursing interventions appropriate for each stage.

2. Ask students to search the Internet for innovative and unusual information about dissociative disorders. Have students bring materials to class, and provide an opportunity to discuss, debunk myths, and critique the media portrayal of these disorders. Identify appropriate content in materials they found.

3. Watch "Three Faces of Eve" and have a discussion about the symptoms and experiences of this woman with dissociative identity disorder.

4. Have students identify common dissociative states (ie, "highway hypnosis," day-dreaming) and talk about what might be occurring psychologically. Relate this discussion to the clinically significant disorders in which this phenomenon plays a major role. Discuss how it might be for the client with dissociative disorder when coping and dealing with his or her illness.

5. Discuss "Type A" personality: its symptoms, difficulty in treating, and association with coronary artery disease.

CHAPTER 22

Personality Development and Personality Disorders

■ Chapter Summary

Personality is the total of one's internal and external patterns of adjustment to life. This chapter discusses theories of personality development; the importance of personality growth and development in the mental health setting; and factors that may contribute to developmental disturbances. Behavioral disturbances are common in personality disorders. There are three groups of personality types: 1) cluster A disorders, with odd, eccentric behavior; 2) cluster B disorders, with emotional, erratic, or dramatic behavior; and 3) cluster C disorders, with anxious and fearful behavior. Culture is important in personality development, and judgments about personality must take into account the individual's ethnic, cultural, and social background. The nursing process includes 1) assessment, including disturbances of cognition, affect, interpersonal functioning, and impulse control that deviate from cultural norms; 2) nursing diagnosis; 3) outcome identification; 4) planning interventions; 5) implementation; and 6) evaluation.

■ Chapter Outline

I. THEORIES OF PERSONALITY DEVELOPMENT
   A. Freud's Psychoanalytic Theory
      Freud's theory describes three major categories: personal development, personality structure, and dynamics of personality. There are three levels of consciousness: unconscious, preconscious (subconscious), and conscious. Organization of personality structure includes id (unconscious reservoir of primitive drives), ego (interacts with outside world), and superego (censoring force or conscience). Dynamics of personality: each person has certain amount of psychic energy to cope. Five phases of the psychobiologic process that have impact on personality: oral, anal, phallic or oedipal, latency, and genital.
   B. Erikson's Psychosocial Theory
      Emphasizes the concept of identity or an inner sense of sameness that perseveres despite changes. Eight psychosocial stages in life,

each having an area of conflict, basic virtues or qualities acquired, and positive and negative behavior.

C. Piaget's Cognitive Developmental Theory
Views intellectual development as result of constant interaction between environment and genetically determined attributes. Four stages of intellectual growth in childhood: sensorimotor, preoperational, concrete operational, formal operational.

II. CAUSES OF PERSONALITY DISORDERS
Healthy personality characterized by positive self-concept, body image, and sense of self-worth; ability to relate openly and honestly. Personality disorder characterized by inflexible, maladaptive behaviors that interfere with functioning. Several factors may predispose to development of personality disorder: 1) biologic predisposition; 2) childhood experiences; 3) social deviance; 4) weak superego; 5) drive for prestige, power; and 6) low degree of social interaction.

III. CHARACTERISTICS OF PERSONALITY DISORDERS
Personality disorder is a nonpsychotic illness characterized by maladaptive behavior. Characteristics of personality disorder are: the person denies maladaptive behaviors; behaviors are inflexible; minor stress is poorly tolerated; person in contact with reality; disturbed mood; and help rarely sought.

IV. DIAGNOSTIC CRITERIA FOR PERSONALITY DISORDERS
A. Cluster A Disorders: Odd, Eccentric Behavior
1. Paranoid Personality Disorder: Chronic hostility projected onto others.
2. Schizoid Personality Disorder: No desire for social involvement, pattern of detachment, restricted range of expression.
3. Schizotypal Personality Disorder: Disturbance in thought processes referred to as magical thinking, superstitiousness, or telepathy, limited social contacts, perceptual disturbances, paranoid ideation.
B. Cluster B Disorders: Emotional, Erratic, or Dramatic Behavior
1. Antisocial Personality Disorder: Sociopathic, psychopathic, and semantic disorders. Conduct disorder is diagnosed if person is under age 18. Symptoms include lack of remorse or indifference to victims, expectation of immediate gratification, failure to accept social norms, impulsivity, irresponsibility, aggression, lying, and reckless behavior.
2. Borderline Personality Disorder: Symptoms include impulsive, unpredictable behavior; inappropriate, intense anger; unstable affect; disturbed self-concept; inability to control one's emotions. Clients report feeling empty, lonely, unable to experience

pleasure. May demonstrate splitting: inability to integrate and accept both positive and negative feelings at the same time. Projective identification can also occur: projecting uncomfortable or aggressive aspects of one's own personality onto external objects.

3. Histrionic Personality Disorder: Pattern of theatrical or overly dramatic behavior; discomfort in situations in which client is not center of attention.

4. Narcissistic Personality Disorder: Exaggerated or grandiose sense of self-importance. Preoccupation with fantasies of success, power; requires excessive admiration; displays arrogance.

C. Cluster C Disorders: Anxious, Fearful Behavior

1. Obsessive–Compulsive Personality Disorder: Obsessive–compulsive traits; preoccupied with rules and regulations; concerned with trivial details; excessively devoted to work and productivity. Depression common.

2. Dependent Personality Disorder: Lacks self-confidence, allows others to become responsible for his or her life.

3. Avoidant Personality Disorder: Sensitive to rejection, criticism, humiliation, disapproval, or shame and appears devastated at slightest amount of disapproval. Anxiety and depression common.

V. TRANSCULTURAL CONSIDERATIONS

Culture is important in personality development. Nurse must be aware of culture's distinctive qualities and variety of lifestyles, values, and structures within it that influence personality development. Judgments about personality must take into account individual's ethnic, cultural, and social background.

VI. THE NURSING PROCESS

A. Assessment

Assess disturbances of cognition, affect, interpersonal functioning, and impulse control that deviate from cultural norms.

1. Disturbance of Cognition: In contact with reality but has difficulty coping with stress. Illusions, depersonalization may be exhibited. Insight and judgment may be impaired.

2. Disturbance of Affect: Assess intensity, degree of lability, and appropriateness of affect.

3. Disturbance of Interpersonal Functioning: Client may be reserved, withdrawn, lonely, or indifferent toward others.

4. Dysfunctional Behavior: Lack of impulse control: assess in structured environment—unpredictable behavior may occur.

B. Nursing Diagnoses
Focus on disturbances of cognition, affect, interpersonal functioning, and impulse control.

C. Outcome Identification
Focus on improving client's ability to differentiate fantasy from reality; develop positive coping skills; improve impulse control; decrease dysfunctional behavior; improve interpersonal relationships; gain increased insight into illness.

D. Planning Interventions
Nurse must have knowledge of personality development and differences in cultural norms; interventions directed at specific behaviors, characteristics, and symptoms common to given disorder.

E. Implementation
Establish accepting environment; specific interventions for disturbances of cognition, affect, interpersonal functioning, and lack of impulse control.
1. Medication Management: Caution is used because clients may not be compliant with medications. History of substance abuse or drug dependency must be assessed.
2. Interactive therapies: Combined extended psychotherapy and medications have been effective. Cognitive behavioral therapy, group therapy, reality therapy, intensive psychoanalysis also used.

F. Evaluation
Can be difficult because of complexity of presentation. Treatment tends to be long term; many clients have recurrent acute episodes.

KEY WORDS

Antisocial	Preconscious
Borderline personality	Projective identification
Conduct disorder	Schizoid
Ego	Schizotypal
Histrionic	Splitting
Id	Superego
Narcissistic	Unconscious

■ Classroom Teaching Strategies

1. Divide the classroom into three groups, assigning each one a cluster (A, B, C) of personality types. Have each group prepare a brief presentation of the various behaviors that are seen in their cluster and provide an example of nursing interventions that would be effective. Encourage

students to be creative and use role-playing, the blackboard, and any other visuals that would assist their classmates to imagine the behaviors.

2. Discuss borderline personality disorder, common symptoms, and nursing interventions. If possible, use film clips (for example, from "Fatal Attraction") to illustrate borderline behaviors. Discuss students' feelings about providing nursing care to someone demonstrating these types of behaviors.

3. Have students think about popular figures, movies, and media. Brainstorm about behaviors that could be symptoms of personality disorder. Discuss what makes symptoms "personality disorders" versus just traits. Use the discussion to highlight issues such as cultural bias, gender bias, and stereotyping in the diagnosis of personality disorder.

4. Ask students to consider which type of personality disorder they might have the most difficulty working with in a clinical setting, and why. Use the discussion to encourage student self-reflection and analysis of personal feelings that may interfere with caring for the individual with personality disorder.

5. Instruct students before class to search the Internet and newspapers for examples of behaviors that might be construed as personality disorder. Discuss how and why this diagnosis might be made, and the factors that would enter into that decision.

CHAPTER 23

Cognitive Disorders

■ Chapter Summary

Cognitive disorders include delirium, dementia (such as Alzheimer's disease), and amnestic disorders. Identifying causes of these disorders is often difficult and confusing. Delirium is the most common and life-threatening of psychiatric illnesses. It is transient, can be acute or subacute in onset, and presents as reversible global dysfunction in cerebral metabolism. Dementia is a form of global or diffuse brain dysfunction characterized by a gradual, progressive, chronic deterioration of intellectual function. Amnestic disorders are characterized by an inability to recall recent or remote events. The nursing process involves assessment of symptoms, behaviors, and cognitive status. Nursing diagnosis and outcome identification are focused around three general goals of care: elimination of organic etiology; prevention of acceleration of symptoms; and preserving the client's dignity. Nursing intervention focuses on preventing injury; promoting adequate physiologic functioning; encouraging expression of feelings; and caring for the client in as nonrestrictive an environment as possible. Caring for clients with cognitive disorders can be challenging, and it is important for the nurse to understand and be aware of his or her own feelings toward aging, cognition, and cultural values.

■ Chapter Outline

I. CAUSES OF COGNITIVE DISORDERS
   Intellect peaks at age 30, plateaus at ages 50 to 60, and then slowly declines until age 70. Memory is not a single homogeneous entity but is composed of four interacting memory systems: working memory; episodic memory; semantic memory; and procedural memory. These systems together contribute to cognitive functioning. The search for the causes of Alzheimer's disease continues. Several theories have been suggested, including genetic theory; immune system theory; oxidation theory; virus and bacteria theory; nutritional theory; and metal deposit theory.

II. CLINICAL SYMPTOMS OF COGNITIVE DISORDERS
   Differentiating delirium from dementia or depression is challenging.

Many of the clinical symptoms overlap, and this can make assessment and diagnosis difficult.

III. DIAGNOSTIC CRITERIA FOR COGNITIVE DISORDERS
  A. Delirium
     The most common and life-threatening psychiatric illness. Transient; can be acute or subacute in onset; presents as reversible global dysfunction in cerebral metabolism. Clinical symptoms: rapid onset; impaired judgment; fluctuating affect and/or mood; recent memory impairment; disorientation; dysnomia (inability to name objects); dysgraphia (impaired ability to write); perceptual disturbances. Restless, agitated behavior. Asterixis (flapping motion of arms) may be seen.
     1. Delirium Due to a General Medical Condition: When cognitive disturbance is the direct physiologic consequence of a general medical condition.
     2. Substance-Induced Delirium: Symptoms occur within minutes or hours of taking relatively high doses of certain drugs.
     3. Delirium Due to Multiple Etiologies: When delirium has more than one etiology.
     4. Delirium Not Otherwise Specified: Does not meet criteria for any other delirium.
  B. Dementia
     A form of global or diffuse brain dysfunction characterized by a gradual, progressive, chronic deterioration of intellectual function. Impaired judgment or inability to make reasonable decisions is one of the earliest signs.
     Symptoms can include disorientation; memory, attention, and concentration deficits; confabulation (filling in memory gaps with false content); perseveration (continued repetition of a behavior); personality change; psychotic disturbance; wandering; suspiciousness; hostility; aggressiveness.
     1. Dementia of the Alzheimer's Type: Alzheimer's disease is the fourth most common cause of death for people older than 65 years in the United States. Symptoms include cognitive deficit; aphasia; apraxia; agnosia; disturbed executive functioning. Several classifications exist to describe the progression of the disorder. One is to group clinical symptoms into three progressive stages: mild, moderate, and severe. Another denotes seven stages of Alzheimer's disease according to functional consequences.
     2. Vascular Dementia
        Second most common cause of dementia after Alzheimer's disease. Onset abrupt with fluctuating, rapid memory changes and other cognitive impairments. Symptoms include apathy, unsteady gait, weakness, dizziness, and sensory loss. Focal

neurologic signs and symptoms include exaggeration of deep tendon reflexes, extensor plantar response; pseudobulbar palsy; gait abnormalities; or weakness of an extremity.
3. Dementia Due to Other General Medical Conditions
Dementias due to medical, endocrine, nutritional, infectious conditions; structural lesions of the brain; and renal or hepatic dysfunction.

C. Amnestic Disorders
Individuals with amnesia are impaired in their ability to recall. Anterograde amnesia is inability to recall events long ago. Retrograde amnesia refers to loss of memory of events occurring before a particular time in the person's life. There are three subtypes of amnestic disorders: amnestic disorder due to general medical condition; substance-induced persisting amnestic disorder; and amnestic disorder not otherwise specified.

D. Cognitive Disorder Not Otherwise Specified: Cognitive dysfunction due to direct physiologic effect of general medical condition that does not meet criteria for any of the other deliriums, dementias, or amnestic disorders

IV. TRANSCULTURAL CONSIDERATIONS
Need to consider client's cultural and educational background when evaluating cognitive capacity; prevalence of dementia varies across cultures; some questions may be culturally bound.

V. THE NURSING PROCESS
A. Assessment
Single most important piece of information is careful history from client's family or another reliable observer. Assessment focuses on severity and duration of cognitive impairment; clinical symptoms; judgment, orientation, memory, affect, and cognition (JOMAC); intellectual ability; appearance and behaviors; comprehensive history and physical; review of medications.

B. Nursing Diagnoses
Six basic commonalities link delirium, dementia, and amnestic disorders: impaired cognition, altered thought process, impaired communication, behavioral disturbances, self-care deficits, and impaired socialization.

C. Outcome Identification
Focus on three general goals of care: elimination of organic etiology; prevention of acceleration of symptoms; and preserving client's dignity.

D. Planning Interventions
Focus on maintaining client's contact with reality; reducing agitation; preventing injury; promoting nutritional and fluid intake;

promoting adequate sleep and rest; encouraging expression of feelings; stimulating memory; decreasing socially inappropriate behavior; encouraging social relationships; using as nonrestrictive an environment as possible.

E. Implementation
Nurse must be aware of personal feelings that can affect care, because caring for the client with delirium and dementia can be challenging.
1. Safe Environment: Use calm, direct, supportive approach with predictable schedule; communicate clearly and simply; minimize stimuli; use "restraint-free environment"; use family members or companion sitters as alternatives to restraint. Goal is to educate caregivers about disease and develop individualized care plan.
2. Medication Management: Common medications include atypical antipsychotics, benzodiazepines, and antidepressants; use with caution to avoid oversedation and adverse reactions.
3. Education: Educate clients, family members, and caregivers about management of clinical symptoms; community support groups. Multidisciplinary approach is optimal.
4. Continuum of care: Vital if client is to have quality of life. Consider hospice care; follow-up contact and bereavement counseling for family members; care in home setting is common.

F. Evaluation
Ongoing process; obtain input from caregivers and family.

KEY WORDS

Agnosia
Alzheimer's disease
Amnestic disorders
Anterograde amnesia
Aphasia
Apraxia
Asterixis
Confabulation
Delirium
Dementia

Dysgraphia
Dysnomia
Focal neurologic signs
Hospice care
JOMAC
Perseveration
Restraint-free environment
Retrograde amnesia
Sundown syndrome

■ Classroom Teaching Strategies

1. Ask students to think about an older person they know who has cognitive deficits. What is the most difficult thing they encountered when interacting with this person? Have students discuss why they might find it challenging to work with the older adult with Alzheimer's disease.

2. Engage students in a discussion about their own aging, their thoughts about it, what they think will be most difficult for them, how they might perceive the older client.

3. On index cards, write down the following words: dysnomia, dysgraphia, asterixis, confabulation, perseveration, aphasia, apraxia, agnosia. Divide the class into pairs and give one index card to each pair. Ask each pair of students to demonstrate the word on their card, and have the remainder of the class try to guess what term and behavior they are demonstrating.

4. Have students brainstorm and write on the chalkboard: "What would it be like not to be able to remember anything about the past?". Focus on feelings and emotional experiences. Use the discussion to enhance the students' empathy for the lived experience of a person with Alzheimer's disease. Discuss ways in which the nurse might be helpful in working with an individual and family having this experience.

5. Have two students come to the front of class to role-play. One student will play the part of the nurse, and one student will play the part of a client with Alzheimer's disease who has become agitated because he or she wants to leave the room and "go back to my home in the country." Use the role-play to demonstrate interventions involving a calm, structured approach, with encouragement and reality testing.

CHAPTER 24

Eating Disorders

■ Chapter Summary

Eating disorders (anorexia nervosa, bulimia nervosa, and obesity) are among the most devastating illnesses confronting the mental health profession. All three disorders may have serious medical complications if left untreated. These disorders are characterized by severe disturbances in eating behavior. Theories of etiology include genetic and biochemical, psychodynamic, and family systems theories. Clinical symptoms include an unhealthy body mass index (BMI), with resulting disturbed physiologic functioning, and unusual thoughts, feelings, and behavior about food. Many cultural variations in eating patterns and beliefs must be considered when working with clients who have eating disorders.

■ Chapter Outline

I. CAUSES
   Theories of eating disorders are characterized as genetic or biochemical, psychodynamic, and family systems theories.

   A. Genetic or Biochemical Theories
      Several theories, including: eating disorders are due to abnormalities in the activity of hormones and neurotransmitters that preserve balance between energy output and food intake; eating disorders are due to high levels of enkephalins and endorphins; anorexia results from hormone imbalance from excessive physical activity; and obsessive-compulsive behaviors are linked with eating disorders.

   B. Psychodynamic Theories
      Hold that the theme of starvation is a form of self-punishment, with the unconscious purpose of pleasing an introjected or internalized parent. Fasting may restore a sense of order and control to a clients. Clients may starve themselves to suppress or control feelings of emotional emptiness, or because they believe parents have not responded adequately to them.

C. Family Systems Theories
Hold that eating disorders result from conflicts between parent and child expectations; family preoccupation with weight and appearance; and enmeshed families.

II. CLINICAL SYMPTOMS

Include unhealthy amount of body fat or BMI and unusual thoughts, feelings, and behavior about food. This may include focus on body weight; constant dieting; impaired body image; preoccupation with food; use of food to satisfy negative feelings; compulsive exercising; fear of not being able to stop eating; abuse of drugs or alcohol; stealing, shoplifting, or prostitution to get money for food.

III. DIAGNOSTIC CRITERIA

A. Anorexia Nervosa
Refusal to maintain normal body weight; fear of weight gain; disturbed perception about the body.

B. Bulimia Nervosa
Episodic binge eating with rapid consumption of large amount of food in less than 2 hours. Client is aware that behavior is abnormal; cannot stop eating voluntarily; and is self-critical.

C. Eating Disorders Not Otherwise Specified
Disorders that do not meet criteria for any other disorder.

IV. OBESITY

Clients with a BMI of 26 to 35 are diagnosed as mildly to moderately obese. Obesity is a physical condition resulting from a medical condition, diet, side effect of medications such as steroids, or compulsive eating that is psychogenic in origin.

V. TRANSCULTURAL CONSIDERATIONS

Anorexia nervosa is prevalent in industrialized societies in which physical attractiveness is linked to being thin. There are many cultural variations in eating patterns and beliefs. Nurse must consider these when working with clients who have eating disorders.

VI. THE NURSING PROCESS

A. Assessment
A complex process; firm but caring approach is helpful; assessment tools can assist the nurse; physical examination is important, including BMI, weight and height, and additional tests, if needed.

B. Nursing Diagnoses
Focus on client's health, nutrition, developmental level, coping skills, emotional status, behavioral responses, and family dynamics.

C. Outcome Identification
Short-term: focus on stabilizing physiology.
Long-term: focus on coping and psychological issues.

D. Planning Interventions
Involve client and family; multidisciplinary approach.

E. Implementation
1. Creating a Safe Environment
Safe, structured environment minimizes potential for injury to self or others. Must assess for suicidal thoughts or other depressive symptoms as behavioral changes and weight gain occur.
2. Stabilizing Medical Condition
Care needed for physical problems and meeting basic client needs. Limit mealtimes; supervision following meals; monitor intake and output, vital signs, weight, activity, lab tests.
3. Stabilizing Behavior
Treatment often based on behavioral methods to stabilize clinical symptoms. Alternate methods may be explored to minimize compulsive exercise habits, such as limit setting.
4. Medication Management
Tricyclic antidepressants, selective serotonin reuptake inhibitors, and opiate antagonist, naltrexone, are effective in stabilizing binging, obsessive-compulsive behavior, and underlying depression. There is a limited role for psychopharmacologic agents in treating anorexia nervosa, although various SSRIs may be of use.
5. Interactive Therapies
Several approaches may be helpful: cognitive behavioral therapy, interpersonal psychotherapy, solution-focused therapy, and family or couple therapy.
6. Self-Help and Support Groups
Can give client information and support during lifelong recovery.
7. Education
Psychoeducational groups are recommended early in treatment. Goal is to provide information and begin correcting erroneous notions about food and eating.

F. Evaluation
Treating eating disorders is time-consuming, emotional, and lengthy; a lifelong process. Evaluating is an ongoing process. Continuum of care includes group therapy, individual therapy, and family therapy.

KEY WORDS
Anorexia nervosa
Body mass index
Bulimia nervosa

Enmeshed family
Lanugo

■ Classroom Teaching Strategies

1. Ask students to search the media and Internet for stories about public figures who have struggled with weight or for which there has been speculation about weight disturbances (for example, Twiggy, Karen Carpenter). Discuss the media portrayal of eating disorders and symptoms that were highlighted. Encourage the students to talk about their perceptions of eating disorders and people who may be experiencing difficulties with eating behaviors.

2. Have students gather data about eating disorders, including prevalence among college students, athletes, and the general public. Discuss the implications of eating disorders as a public health issue. Talk about ways that young women could be educated to avoid focusing on weight and appearance.

3. Ask students to get newspaper clippings and magazine ads that focus on thinness, dieting, and the view of women as objects. Discuss how these social mores and values might influence young women; problem-solve about ways this might be addressed in our society.

4. Present a case study of an anorexic college student, including symptoms and history of eating behaviors. Ask students to develop a care plan, focusing on assessment, nursing diagnosis, and intervention during an acute hospitalization.

5. Have students search the media and Internet for stories or reports about obesity. Compare and contrast these with those found about anorexia/bulimia. What are the differences in the ways in which the media portray obesity compared to anorexia?

6. Have students compare and contrast anorexia nervosa with bulimia nervosa, including theories of etiology and the symptomatology of each disorder.

CHAPTER 25

Substance-Related Disorders

■ Chapter Summary

There is a high incidence of drug and alcohol abuse among all age groups in America. This chapter presents a comprehensive overview of substance abuse, including drugs, alcohol, nicotine, and caffeine. Theories about substance abuse include biologic and genetic, learning theories, and social theories. The disease concept of alcoholism is discussed, including clinical symptoms and behaviors and physiological effects of a variety of substances. Alcohol-related disorders and alcohol-induced disorders are presented. The symptoms and treatments for other substances include drugs such as sedatives, hypnotics, anxiolytics, opioids, amphetamines, cocaine, cannabis, hallucinogens, phencyclidine, inhalants, caffeine, and nicotine. The nursing process is focused on assessment, nursing diagnoses, outcome identification, treatment planning, implementation, and evaluation.

■ Chapter Outline

I. ALCOHOL USE AND ABUSE

Abuse of alcohol is a major health problem for several million Americans, including children, adults, and adolescents. Risky drinking patterns result in serious alcohol-related problems, including traumatic or fatal injuries from motor vehicle accidents, drowning, burns, severe depression, suicide, or homicide.

II. SUBSTANCE USE AND ABUSE

The use of illicit drugs has escalated across the country, and most illicit users have long histories of drug use. The development of addiction after young adulthood is rare. Both alcoholism and substance abuse are responsible for dysfunctional marital and family relationships, divorce, desertion, child abuse, displaced children, and impoverished families.

III. CAUSES OF ADDICTION

A. Biologic and Genetic Theories

The discovery that all drugs of abuse have one thing in common— namely, the stimulation of dopamine secretion—occurred in the

1980s. With the use of scientific innovations, studies have identified the neural structures and pathways responsible for pleasure and reinforcement of behavior. Some individuals have a predisposition to or are at risk for addiction due to a high level of stress hormones, a deficit in dopamine function that is temporarily connected to their drug of choice, or a genetically based phenomenon in the brains of people at risk for alcoholism.

B. Learning Theory
    Behavioral theorists believe that addiction is the result of the positive effect of mood alterations that one experiences using drugs or alcohol. The brain is specifically designed to absorb and respond in very powerful ways to environmental cues and contexts, such as large doses of mind-altering drugs.

C. Social Theories
    A drug must be available in sufficient amounts to sustain addiction. Teenagers are at risk for alcohol abuse because it is the drug of choice among most adults, it is legal, and it is socially acceptable. Teens are also at risk for substance abuse as they possess more leisure time and money and experience less parental or community supervision.

D. The Addictive Personality
    Many theorists consider individuals who abuse substances to be fixed at an oral or infantile level of development. Characteristics seen include low self-esteem, feelings of dependency, low tolerance for frustration and anxiety, antisocial behavior, and fear. Other theories involve beliefs about early childhood rejection, overprotection, or undue responsibility.

E. Disease Concept of Alcoholism
    Most authorities in the field of alcohol abuse base their beliefs on the pioneer work of Jellinick (1960), who surveyed and classified alcoholics into five types and also identified four progressive phases that the alcoholic experiences. Tolerance occurs as the individual drinks more with a decreased effect; withdrawal occurs when an individual abruptly stops drinking after alcohol has become a necessity for maintaining functioning. Alcoholism can be fatal.

IV. CLINICAL SYMPTOMS OF SUBSTANCE-RELATED DISORDERS
     Substance-dependent individuals often exhibit similar clinical symptoms, including impaired judgment, orientation, memory, affect, and cognition; impaired speech; behavioral changes; and impaired mobility.

V. DIAGNOSTIC CRITERIA FOR ALCOHOL-RELATED DISORDERS
    There are two categories for alcohol-related disorders: alcohol use disorders (including alcohol dependence and alcohol abuse) and alcohol-induced disorders (includes 12 subtypes).

A. Alcohol Use Disorders
   1. Alcohol Dependence
      Essential feature: a cluster of cognitive, behavioral, and physiologic symptoms indicating that the individual continues use of alcohol despite critical alcohol-related problems.
   2. Alcohol Abuse
      One or more of the following in a 12-month period: recurrent drinking of alcohol resulting in failure to fulfill major roles; recurrent drinking in situations in which it is physically hazardous; recurrent alcohol-related legal problems; continued use despite having persistent or recurrent social or interpersonal problems caused by alcoholism.
B. Alcohol-Induced Disorders
   1. Alcohol Intoxication
      Occurs after recently ingesting alcohol; behavioral changes such as impaired occupational or social functioning, fighting, impaired judgment.
   2. Alcohol Withdrawal
      Occurs within several hours to a few days after cessation or reduction in heavy and prolonged drinking; symptoms of autonomic hyperactivity; increased hand tremor; sleep disturbances, insomnia, or nightmares; nausea or vomiting; transient visual, tactile, auditory hallucinations or illusions; psychomotor agitation; anxiety; and grand mal seizures.
   3. Alcohol Withdrawal Delirium
      Called delirium tremens; may occur within 24 to 72 hours after last drink; elevated vital signs; restlessness; tremulousness; agitation; hyperalertness; illusions, hallucinations.
   4. Alcohol-Induced Persisting Dementia
      Severe loss of intellectual ability that interferes with social or occupational functioning; impaired memory, judgment, and abstract thinking.
   5. Alcohol-Induced Persisting Amnestic Disorder
      Two nervous system disorders associated with poor nutritional habits after long-term alcohol use: Korsakoff's psychosis (amnesia characterized by loss of short-term memory) and Wernicke's encephalopathy (inflammatory hemorrhagic, degenerative brain condition caused by thiamine deficiency).
   6. Other Alcohol-Induced Disorders
      Include depression, anxiety, sexual dysfunction, sleep disorders.

VI. EFFECTS OF ALCOHOL
   Numerous physiologic effects, including gastrointestinal tract complications; cardiovascular system complications; respiratory tract complications; reproductive system complications; fetal alcohol

syndrome during pregnancy; central nervous system depression; peripheral neuropathy; gait changes; nerve palsy.

VII. DIAGNOSTIC CRITERIA FOR OTHER SUBSTANCE-RELATED DISORDERS

"Addiction" is a term used to define a state of chronic or recurrent drug intoxication, characterized by psychological and physical dependence as well as tolerance.

A. Sedative-, Hypnotic-, or Anxiolytic-Related Disorders
Substances: benzodiazepines; carbamates; barbiturates; barbiturate-like hypnotics; prescription sleeping medication; and all anxiolytic medications. Barbiturates—leading cause of accidental poisoning and primary method of committing suicide.

B. Opioid-Related Disorders
Opioids: resemble opium or alkaloid derivatives; opiate: any chemical derived from opium. Both are narcotic drugs that induce sleep, suppress coughing, and alleviate pain; considered the most addictive drugs. Withdrawal symptoms begin 12 to 16 hours after last dose.

C. Amphetamine-Related Disorders
Amphetamines: "pep pills"; directly stimulate central nervous system; create feeling of alertness and self-confidence. Effects on the body: increased heart rate; elevated blood pressure; excitability; hand tremors; talkativeness; diaphoresis; dry mouth; abnormal heart rhythms; headaches; pallor; diarrhea; unclear speech.

D. Cocaine-Related Disorders
Cocaine: stimulant substance. Common physical effects: pupillary dilation; increased blood pressure, respirations, and temperature; less common effects: loss of appetite, insomnia, impaired thinking, agitation, panic attacks or cocaine psychosis.

E. Cannabis-Related Disorders
Marijuana is the most widely used illegal drug. Physical effects: increased appetite, lowered body temperature, depression, drowsiness, unsteady gait, inability to think clearly, excitement, reduced coordination and reflexes. Not physically addictive, but can lead to psychological dependence.

F. Hallucinogen- and Phencyclidine-Related Disorders
Hallucinogens and PCP associated with abuse because physiologic dependence has not been demonstrated. Dangerous; can lead to panic, paranoia, flashbacks, or death. Symptoms: increased vital signs; dilated pupils; hand tremors; cold, sweaty palms; flushed face; irregular respirations; nausea. Unpredictable effects; PCP especially is dangerous; intoxication results in feelings of enormous strength, paranoia, and no feelings of pain.

G. Inhalant-Related Disorders
Inhalants: chemicals that give off fumes or vapors when inhaled.
Cause confusion, excitement, hallucinations. Commonly abused
inhalants: glue, gasoline, lighter fluid, paint thinner, varnish,
shellac, nail polish remover, aerosol-packaged products.

H. Caffeine- and Nicotine-Related Disorders
Some people show clinical symptoms of dependence, tolerance, and
withdrawal when consuming large amounts of caffeine. Nicotine: a
stimulant that elevates blood pressure and increases heart rate.

VIII. DESIGNER DRUGS AND STEROIDS
Designer drugs: manufactured in clandestine labs and made available
on the street. Potent reinforcers and addictive.

IX. TRANSCULTURAL CONSIDERATIONS
Wide cultural variations in attitudes toward substance consumption,
patterns of use, accessibility, physiologic reactions, prevalence of
substance abuse disorders.

X. THE NURSING PROCESS
A. Assessment
Data collection must be comprehensive and done systematically.
1. Alcohol
Several screening tests are available for alcohol assessment,
including the Michigan Alcohol Screening Test (MAST), the
CAGE Screening Test for Alcoholism, and the Alcohol Use
Disorders Identification Test (AUDIT). Diagnostic laboratory
tests may also be needed, in addition to neurologic evaluation
and psychiatric consultation.
2. Substances Other Than Alcohol
Clients who abuse substances present challenges to assessment.
Direct questions toward substance identification; amount and
frequency of use; duration of use; route of administration;
history of suicidal ideation or attempts; withdrawal symptoms;
longest drug-free period; and desire for treatment. The nurse
must recognize symptoms of and potential for withdrawal or
overdose during the assessment process.

B. Nursing Diagnoses
Diagnoses identify health needs requiring nursing intervention.
Clients may have poor general health and inadequate nutrition;
more susceptible to infections and medical complications; potential
for injury; impaired communication and social interaction.

C. Outcome Identification
Outcome criteria focus on providing a safe environment; stabilizing
existing medical problems; improving impaired cognition and

communication; establishing nutritious eating patterns; balancing rest, sleep, activity; developing alternative coping skills; resolving personal and family issues related to disorder.

D. Planning Interventions
Multidisciplinary and comprehensive. An "intervention" is an organized, deliberate confrontation of a client who uses or abuses substances; staged to overcome denial; recognize that help is available; and seek help.

E. Implementation
General approaches include maintaining one-to-one contacts; orienting client to reality; speaking slowly and clearly; avoiding judgment; offering support.
   1. Safe Environment
      Safety is priority due to possibility of symptoms of overdose, intoxication, or withdrawal. Reduce stimuli; monitor symptoms; institute seizure precautions.
   2. Stabilization of Medical Condition
      Promote adequate nutrition and hydration; check vital signs; observe for current or impending delirium tremens; monitor intake and output; evaluate for intravenous therapy; monitor cardiac status; lab tests as appropriate.
   3. Stabilization of Behavior
      Clients often manipulative; drug-seeking; antipsychotics may be needed.
   4. Medication Management
      Use caution with substance abusers. Benzodiazepines or intravenous barbiturates used for delirium tremens.
   5. Disulfiram and Naltrexone Therapy
      Aversion therapy: giving a drug such as emetine and then following it with alcohol, which induces nausea and vomiting. Disulfiram (Antabuse) interferes with alcohol breakdown. Naltrexone (ReVia) reduces craving and blocks alcohol's effects.
   6. Interactive Therapies
      Individual psychotherapy, group therapy, family therapy can be effective. Codependency: living in shadow of another person's chemical dependency.
   7. Smoking Cessation Programs
      Nicotine replacement therapy and behavior modification are common approaches to help clients stop smoking.
   8. Support and Self-Help Groups
      Several types available for clients who want treatment.

F. Evaluation
Evaluation is dynamic and incorporates alternative strategies, based on ongoing and systematic evaluation. Continuum of care is difficult and costly.

KEY WORDS

Addiction

Addictive personality

Amphetamines

Cannabis

Cocaine

Fetal alcohol syndrome

Hallucinogens

Korsakoff's psychosis

Opioid

PCP

Psychosis

Tolerance

Wernicke's encephalopathy

Withdrawal

■ Classroom Teaching Strategies

1. Assign several groups in class to one group of substances. Have students describe the substance; its mechanism of action on the brain; its physiologic effects on the body; and behaviors and symptoms that result from abuse of the substance.

2. Ask students to consider and discuss "the user's view" of substance use and abuse, including reasons for using, desired effects from using, and why an individual may not want to stop using.

3. Ask students to think about cultural issues that are operant in contemporary American society, and how cultures may differ in their "group consciousness" about addictive disorders.

4. Have students discuss the phenomenon of delirium tremens (DTs), focusing on nursing assessment, interventions, and critical safety issues in treating the client at risk for DTs. Ask students to develop a protocol for assessment and management of DTs in the inpatient medical setting.

5. Stage an "intervention" during class. Have students act out the roles of a substance user, the user's significant other, and various other family members (children, aunts, uncles, grandparents, and so forth). Use the role-playing as a springboard for talking about the feelings and perspectives of each person and the issues that may be relevant for each.

CHAPTER 26

Sexual Disorders

■ Chapter Summary

Sex is one of four primary drives that also include thirst, hunger, and avoidance of pain. Sexual acts occur when behaviors involve genitalia and erogenous zones. Sexuality is the result of several factors that shape an individual's self-perception, feelings of attractiveness, sensuality, pleasure, and affirmation of one's gender identity. Nurses come into contact with a variety of client concerns regarding sexual identity or activity. Self-awareness is important to understanding and discussing sexual issues with clients. Gender identity develops as a result of physiologic, psychosocial, and cultural factors. There are a number of sexual dysfunctions, and this chapter provides a summary and overview of each. The nursing process focuses on assessing the nature and extent of the sexual difficulty; diagnosis and outcome identification evolve from the assessment process. Interventions are individualized based on the client's sexual concern or disorder, causative factors, and clinical symptoms, and focus on the client's specific problems or complaints, respecting his or her cultural and religious preferences. Evaluation is an important component of the nursing process.

■ Chapter Outline

I. THEORIES OF GENDER IDENTITY DEVELOPMENT

   A. Genetic and Biologic Theories
   The male sperm cell determines the sex of the embryo at conception; an X and Y chromosome combination produces a male; two X chromosomes produce a female. Klinefelter's syndrome occurs in males as a result of XXY chromosome grouping; low testosterone levels, small testes, infertility, low sexual interest. Turner's syndrome occurs in females as a result of missing sex chromosome or XO grouping; short stature, lack functional gonads. Gender identity continually evolves under the influence of androgens. Pseudohermaphrodites are individuals who are declared female at birth and are raised as girls but who have a testosterone surge and gender confusion as they approach adolescence. Ambiguous genitalia: penis and small vaginal opening.

B. Psychosocial Theories
Recent theories have explored the impact of gender, race, and ethnicity on gender identity. Gender identity is shaped by attitudes, values, beliefs, sex roles, religious values, family and ethnic communities, and degree of acculturation. Psychosocial aspects of gender identity development include average age of "coming out," self-identity as lesbian/gay, and sharing sexual identity with others.

II. DEVELOPMENT OF SEXUALITY
A. Infancy and Childhood
Age-related developmental stages are related to sexuality and gender orientation.
B. Preadolescence and Adolescence
Children experience sexual feelings, exhibit sexual interest, and undergo sexual body changes as they develop interpersonal relationships.
C. Adulthood
Mature relationships with peers established. Expressions of sexuality may vary as the individual continues to work through developmental stages of middle adulthood and late adulthood or maturity. Sexuality is a human force throughout life and during the dying process. Nurses should encourage the client and family to discuss sexual issues and needs.

III. HUMAN SEXUAL RESPONSE CYCLE
Phases include desire, excitement, orgasm, and resolution.

IV. DIAGNOSTIC CRITERIA FOR SEXUAL DISORDERS
A. Sexual Dysfunctions
Characteristics include disturbances in the sexual response cycle or pain during sexual intercourse.
1. Sexual Desire Disorders: Hypoactive sexual desire disorder is diagnosed only if lack of desire causes distress to client or partner. Sexual aversion disorder involves anxiety, fear, disgust when confronted with a sexual opportunity.
2. Sexual Arousal Disorders: Female: may experience little or no subjective sense of arousal. Male erectile disorder: inability to attain or maintain an erection adequate for sexual activity.
3. Orgasmic Disorders: Recurrent persistent inhibited orgasm following adequate sexual excitement phase, in absence of any organic cause. Premature ejaculation: ejaculation before the person wishes owing to absence of reasonable voluntary control during the sexual response.
4. Sexual Pain Disorders: Dyspareunia: recurrent, persistent genital pain in the male or female. Vaginismus: recurrent and persistent spasms of musculature of vagina that interfere with sexual act.

5. Sexual Dysfunction Due to a General Medical Condition:
   Presence of clinically significant sexual dysfunction that is due to
   the direct physiologic effects of a general medical condition,
   causing marked distress or interpersonal difficulty during sexual
   activity.

B. Paraphilias
   Disorders in which unusual or bizarre sexual imagery or acts are
   enacted to achieve sexual excitement; not usually brought to
   attention of health professionals unless behaviors create conflict
   with society. Features of persons with paraphilias include emotional
   immaturity, fear of sexual relations, shyness, low or poor self-
   concept, depression.

C. Gender Identity Disorders
   Strong and persistent cross-gender identification in which one
   expresses desire or insistence to be of the opposite sex.

V. SEXUAL ADDICTION

Engaging in obsessive-compulsive sexual behavior that causes severe
stress to addicted individuals and their families.

VI. TRANSCULTURAL CONSIDERATIONS

Ethnic, cultural, religious, and social background influences sexual
attitude, desire, and expectations. What is considered deviant behavior
in one cultural setting may be acceptable in another.

VII. THE NURSING PROCESS

A. Assessment
   To take a sexual history, provide a nonthreatening, quiet, private
   environment. Approach subject with professionalism, provide
   support without judgment, and use simple words and phrases. Four
   common barriers: 1) not seeing sexual history as relevant; 2)
   inadequate training; 3) embarrassment of health care professional;
   4) fear of offending client.

B. Nursing Diagnoses
   Sexual Dysfunction diagnosis used when client experiences or is at
   risk of experiencing a change in sexual function that is viewed as
   unrewarding or inadequate, client's verbalization of problem with
   sexual function, or report of limited sexual performance. Rape
   Trauma Syndrome is experienced as a result of forced, violent
   sexual assault against one's will and without one's consent.

C. Outcome Identification
   Outcomes related to sexual function should be made with the input
   of the client, even though they are very personal.

D. Planning Interventions
   Focuses on client's specific problems or complaints, respecting his or her cultural and religious preferences. Planned to meet client's basic human needs, provide structured and protective care, and explore ways to rechannel into sexually acceptable behavior.

E. Implementation
   Interventions are individualized based on client's sexual concern or disorder, causative factors, and clinical symptoms.
   1. Meeting Basic Human Needs: Adequate rest, exercise, nutrition, and good general physical health promote sexual health.
   2. Providing a Safe Environment: Safety is a priority. Environmental manipulation has been effective in relieving anxiety and altering the undesirable behavior of sex offenders.
   3. Medication Management: Various pharmacologic approaches are used to treat clients with sexual disorders; nurse must be aware of applications and potential side effects.
   4. Medical Management: Nurse's role varies depending on setting in which client is assessed and treated. Nurses use biologic interventions when providing care.
   5. Interactive Therapies
      a. Individual Psychotherapy: Recommended for clients who have had a recent life change; clients should be encouraged to seek counseling for themselves and their partners.
      b. Marital Therapy: Marital therapy or counseling effective in managing conflicts, especially if couple has differing opinions or points of view.
      c. Family Therapy: Provides education, information, and support; helps parents learn to cope with and accept adolescent's sexual identity.
      d. Sex Therapy: Provided by trained and certified individuals.
   6. Support Groups: A variety of organizations offer support groups regarding issues of sexuality and sexual health.
   7. Education: Can begin with explanation of normal sexual response; can include explanations about natural changes in sexual function with aging.

F. Evaluation
   Important because outcomes are based on client's expectations. Evaluation focuses on whether the client's expectations are realistic and whether the client feels the need to continue with supportive therapy.

KEY WORDS

Ambiguous genitalia

Coming out

Dyspareunia

Gender identity

Klinefelter's syndrome

Paraphilias

Premature ejaculation

Pseudohermaphrodites

Rape trauma syndrome

Sex

Sexual acts

Sexual addiction

Sexuality

Turner's syndrome

Vaginismus

■ Classroom Teaching Strategies

1. Discuss the difference between the terms *sex, sexuality,* and *sexual acts.*

2. Invite a speaker from a local rape crisis center to come to class and present the services offered by rape crisis and the importance of providing these services. Ask students to explore what types of rape crisis services are available to them locally.

3. Have students consider their opinions and feelings about sexuality and assessing sexuality in their clients. Describe common feelings and ways to deal with them.

4. Have students discuss the importance of sexual assessment and the role of cultural and societal values in the area of sexual functioning and sexuality.

5. Have students identify the four blocks to obtaining a sexual history, and provide examples of these blocks in action. Then, identify at least two ways in which the student might work toward overcoming these obstacles in his or her practice.

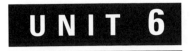

UNIT 6

Special Populations

CHAPTER 27

Infant, Child, and Adolecent Clients

■ Chapter Summary

Diagnosing and treating childhood psychiatric disorders is not an easy task. The etiology of mental and emotional disorders is multifactorial; that is, there is no single causal agent. This chapter focuses on disorders of infancy, childhood, and adolescence, which usually occur as a result of complex reactions during one's early developmental stages. Theories of etiology are discussed, including biologic and genetic theories, psychosocial, and environmental factors. A review of clinical syndromes is provided. Transcultural issues include the fact that intelligence testing should reflect adequate attention to ethnic or cultural background to avoid a misdiagnosis such as mental retardation. The environment, including social and economic context, should be assessed prior to making diagnoses. Treatment is multifaceted and focuses on the needs and problems of the client and family. The nursing process is reviewed, including assessment, diagnosis, outcome identification, planning interventions, and evaluation of the effectiveness of biologic and psychosocial treatments.

■ Chapter Outline

I. CAUSES
   A. Genetic/Biologic Theories
      1. Attention Deficit/Hyperactivity Disorder (ADHD)
         Study of the genetics of behavioral disorders has been limited because of the overlap between one or more syndromes, such as depression, anxiety, enuresis, or a tic disorder. ADHD is a heterogeneous behavioral disorder with multiple etiologies.
      2. Pervasive Developmental Disorders
         The gene has been found for Rett's disorder, an X-linked progressive neurodevelopmental disorder that is one of the most common causes of mental retardation in girls. Down syndrome is a common form of mental retardation caused by a chromosomal abnormality. Other developmental disorders have been linked to a variety of other traumas suffered by fetuses (radiation, alcohol, or drugs in utero, for example).

3. Conduct Disorder
   The most important contributors to conduct disorder are brain abnormalities and atrophy, which have been confirmed by magnetic resonance imaging and electroencephalography.
4. Childhood Psychosis
   Although there is a genetic component, this alone does not explain the development of childhood schizophrenia. Early-onset schizophrenia encompasses a spectrum of disorders due to neuropathology. Other factors, such as intrauterine stress, communication style, life events, and stress are etiologic factors as well. Biologic factors include genetics, neuropathology, and neurotransmitter abnormalities.
5. Autistic Disorder
   Many idiopathic autism cases appear to be an inherited form of an affective disorder.

B. Psychosocial Factors
   1. Children in Families With Conflict or Divorce
      Children are often scapegoated in families, receiving the angry, hostile, frustrated, or ambivalent emotions experienced by various family members. Abnormal family roles are created for children when too much responsibility is placed on them.
   2. Children Who Experience Poverty
      Children in poverty are usually denied access to health care, child care, nutrition, and adequate housing, school, and play environments.
   3. Children of Minority Ethnic Status
      Minority children often experience adverse effects related to their ethnicity because of the existence of poverty and racism.
   4. Children Who Are Abused
      Child abuse can be physical, emotional, or sexual. Abuse places children at risk for various emotional and behavioral disorders and can result in death.
   5. Children of Substance-Abusing and Mentally Ill Parents
      The terms "crack babies" and "fetal alcohol syndrome" describe the effects of maternal crack addiction and alcoholism on children. Children of mentally ill parents are often neglected.
   6. Children of Teenage Parents
      Parenting skills of teens are often insufficient to deal with the stressors of family life. These children are at risk for developmental disorders, behavior or conduct disorders, and emotional problems.
   7. Children With Chronic Illness or Disability
      Children are at risk for psychiatric disorders if they have a chronic medical condition or disability.

C. Environmental Factors
   School environments can influence the development of normal,

positive behavior in children. In addition, neighborhoods can also influence the development of behavior disorders.

II. CLASSIFICATION OF CLINICAL DISORDERS

A. Mental Retardation

Mental retardation is described as the presence of subaverage general intellectual functioning (IQ of approximately 70 or below), associated with or resulting in impairments in adaptive behavior.

B. Pervasive Developmental Disorders

1. Autistic Disorder

Incurable, a lifelong disability. Characterized by qualitative impairments in communication; withdrawal; gross deficits in language development; restricted repetitive and stereotyped patterns of behavior, interest, and activities; and inability to establish meaningful relationships.

2. Asperger's Disorder

Part of the mild end of the autistic spectrum; child has normal or higher intelligence, is clumsy, has poor handwriting, and exhibits autistic-type behavior such as hand flapping or pacing when excited or upset.

C. Attention Deficit and Disruptive Behavior Disorders

1. ADHD

Characteristics include short attention span, impulsivity, distractibility; stubbornness; negativism; temper tantrums; obstinacy; poor self-image; and aggressiveness.

2. Conduct Disorder

The largest single group of psychiatric illnesses in adolescents. Multiple symptoms; symptoms develop first within family unit when child attempts to cope with anxiety or resolve an inner conflict; usually unstable or poor interpersonal relationships within family.

D. Tic Disorders

Tic is a rapid, largely involuntary movement or noise. Can be motor tics (rapid movement of a muscle) or vocal tics (simple throat clearing to more complex vocalizations). Chronic tic disorder involves the presence of either motor or vocal tics, but not both. Tourette's syndrome (Gilles de la Tourette's syndrome) is a combination of motor tics and involuntary vocal and verbal utterances that are often obscene.

E. Elimination Disorders

Enuresis (repeated urination, day or night, into bed or clothes) or encopresis (fecal soiling). Child may be poorly cared for, under stress, experiencing increased anxiety, immature, regressed, or mentally retarded.

F. Other Disorders of Infancy, Childhood, or Adolescence
1. Separation Anxiety Disorder
May develop after some life stress. Consists of excessive anxiety when child is separated from the parent, a significant other, the home, or familiar surroundings. Symptoms (headache, nausea, vomiting, stomachache) seen frequently when child anticipates separation or when actually separated.

G. Mood Disorders: Childhood and Adolescent Depression
Disorders resembling adult depression can and do occur in childhood. There is a familial link. Symptoms of childhood depression include sadness; withdrawal; irritable, negative behavior; low self-esteem; excessive guilt; sleep disturbance; running-away behavior; change in appetite; somatic or physical complaints; difficulty in school; preoccupation with death. Symptoms of adolescent depression include sadness; anger, rage, verbal sarcasm and attack; overreaction to criticism; guilt; poor self-esteem; loss of confidence; hopelessness or helplessness; ambivalence; emptiness; restlessness and agitation; pessimism about future; death wishes, suicidal thoughts or plans or attempts; appetite and sleep disturbances.

H. Adjustment Disorder of Childhood and Adolescence
Maladaptive reaction is in response to an identifiable event or situation that is stress-producing and is not the result or part of a mental disorder.

III. TRANSCULTURAL CONSIDERATIONS
Intelligence testing should reflect adequate attention to ethnic or cultural background to avoid a misdiagnosis such as mental retardation. The environment, including social and economic context, should be assessed prior to making diagnoses.

IV. THE NURSING PROCESS
A. Assessment
Often complicated in young persons by interaction of psychopathology with child's environment and with developmental processes. Medical history, physical and neurologic examinations, lab testing, and psychoeducational testing may be needed. Information needed from teachers, parent, or adult caretakers. Play therapy often used.

B. Nursing Diagnoses
Nursing diagnosis is based on client's problems, strengths, coping abilities, adaptiveness of the symptoms, and inferences about the etiology of the specific disorder.

C. Outcome Identification
Outcomes usually focus on a reduction of clinical symptoms,

decreased stress, progression of normal developmental stages, and therapeutic changes.

D. Planning and Implementing Interventions
Planning interventions is a collaborative effort with client and parents; may require involvement of other disciplines or community supports. Treatment is based on the needs and problems of the client and family. Nursing interventions include helping child master developmental tasks; establishing communication; identifying stimuli that may foster abusive or negative behavior; and allowing time for client to respond to interventions.
  1. Mental Retardation
  Clients may be educable or trainable; may require custodial care.
  2. ADHD
  Multifactorial approach is most effective.
  3. Conduct Disorder
  Interventions focus on maintaining safety and helping child develop internal limits, problem-solving skills, and self-responsibility for acts of antisocial behavior.
  4. Autistic Disorder
  Considered the most irreversible childhood disorder; difficult to treat. Determining most effective mode of communication is important; speak calmly; allow client adequate time to respond; provide safe, consistent environment; behavior management.
  5. Childhood and Adolescent Depression
  Nursing interventions are similar to those for adult clients: provide a safe and therapeutic environment; develop therapeutic relationship; help verbalize feelings (play or art therapy is useful); monitor antidepressant medication and side effects.

E. Continuum of Care
  1. Hospitalization
  2. Day hospitals
  3. Alternative families
  4. Individual psychotherapy
  5. Family therapy (systems therapy)
  6. Group therapy
  7. Play therapy
  8. Behavioral therapy
  9. Art and music therapy

F. Evaluation
An ongoing process. Consider developmental stage of client and whether changes in mood or behavior have occurred since initial assessment. Evaluate efficacy of prescribed medication; family dynamics; and socialization and progress in school.

KEY WORDS

Asperger's disorder
Attention deficit/hyperactivity
    disorder (ADHD)
Autistic disorder
Crack babies
Down syndrome

Encopresis
Enuresis
Fetal alcohol syndrome
Rett's disorder
Scapegoat
Tourette's syndrome

■ Classroom Teaching Strategies

1. Have students prepare a comprehensive care plan for a child with Down syndrome. Include the physiologic, emotional, and social needs of the client and family. Have students also provide a brief overview of the syndrome, including behaviors and symptoms.

2. Ask students to search the Internet for sites that relate to ADHD. Sort out the variety of sites by the information provided and the accuracy of the material presented. Try to find sites that do not provide accurate data about the syndrome, and ask students to critique them. Have students include some sites that give only lay information from individuals who are dealing with ADHD in themselves or in a child.

3. Ask two groups of students to prepare 15-minute presentations on crack babies and fetal alcohol syndrome. Have students compare and contrast the symptoms and clinical nursing care of babies with these two disorders. Engage the class in a discussion of the complexity of these infant disorders, including social and psychological issues.

4. Provide students with a vignette about a 12-year-old girl diagnosed with conduct disorder. Present psychosocial data, symptomatology, and behaviors exhibited. Ask students to discuss the various factors that might be affecting the child's diagnosis; include nursing interventions for each. Discuss nursing interventions for selected problematic behaviors (such as not following rules, angry outbursts, and so forth).

5. Engage the class in a discussion of why infant, childhood, and adolescent disorders are often underdiagnosed and treated in America. What factors contribute to this? What is the cost of this lack of treatment in regard to society? Use the discussion to highlight the social, political, cultural, and economic issues involved in providing mental health care to people in general and to young persons specifically.

CHAPTER 28

Suicidal Clients

■ Chapter Summary

Many Americans have been affected by suicide. In the United States, suicide is the eighth leading cause of death. Causes can range from biologic factors (such as genetic links and neurotransmitter function) to psychosocial factors (such as life events, clients' feelings and emotions, and isolation). This chapter reviews populations who are at high risk for suicide, such as clients with psychiatric and/or neurologic disorders, clients with alexithymia, medically ill clients, adolescents, the elderly, and homosexuals. The nursing process is reviewed, including assessment (an ongoing process, during which the nurse must establish a therapeutic relationship and encourage verbalization of negative feelings), nursing diagnoses, outcome identification, planning, implementation, and evaluation. The role of the nurse in the treatment and prevention of suicide is discussed, as well as the importance of postvention for suicide survivors. Euthanasia and physician-assisted suicide are presented as variants of self-destructive and suicidal ideation and behaviors.

■ Chapter Outline

I. CAUSES

   A. Biologic Theories

      There is a genetic marker for suicidal ideation (a 5-HT2a receptor gene allele C of 102T/C polymorphism). Research has focused on the relationship between serotonin and postsynaptic frontal cortices' binding sites, 5-HIAA, and serum cholesterol.

   B. Psychosocial Factors

      Several causative psychosocial factors have been identified, including: failure to adapt; feelings of alienation or isolation; anger or hostility; reunion wish or fantasy; a way to end one's feelings of hopelessness and helplessness; a cry for help; an attempt to "save face" or seek release to a better life.

II. INDIVIDUALS AT RISK FOR SELF-DESTRUCTIVE BEHAVIOR

   Approximately 80% of those persons attempting suicide give clues, including: verbal clues, behavioral clues, or situational clues.

A. Clients with a Psychiatric Disorder
Among the most serious risk factors are those of various psychiatric disorders, such as major depression, schizophrenia, schizoaffective disorder, bipolar disorder, personality disorders, eating disorders, and alcoholism or drug abuse.

B. Clients with Alexithymia
Alexithymia is a term used to characterize persons who seem not to understand the feelings they experience, and who seem to lack the words to describe their feelings to others. Individuals who experience this phenomenon have been found to be at higher risk for self-mutilation and suicidal behaviors.

C. Clients with a Neurologic Disorder
The presence of neurologic disorders (such as multiple sclerosis, Huntington's, epilepsy, traumatic brain injury, and spinal cord injury) raises the overall suicide risk.

D. Clients With a Medical Illness
Individuals with chronic or terminal medical illnesses have verbalized several reasons for suicidal ideation: pain, suffering, fatigue, loss of independence, and decreased quality of life.

E. High-Risk Populations
High-risk populations include adolescents, ethnic minorities, homosexuals, and the elderly.

F. Other Groups
Individuals whose occupations require selfless public service and dedication and who work under pressure are at risk for suicide.

III. TRANSCULTURAL CONSIDERATIONS
There is little information available about cultural beliefs about suicide. In some cultures, culturally sanctioned suicide exists. In others, suicide is forbidden.

IV. THE NURSING PROCESS
A. Assessment
Suicide is considered more preventable than any other cause of death. Assessment includes applying close observational and listening skills to detect any suicide clues, plan, and degree of lethality. Some terms used to describe the range of suicidal thoughts and behaviors are: suicidal ideation; suicidal intent; suicidal threat; suicidal gesture; intentional self-destructive behavior. Assessment is an ongoing process, during which the nurse must establish a therapeutic relationship and encourage verbalization of negative feelings. There are many scales that may be useful in the assessment process.

B. Nursing Diagnoses
Diagnosis is based on the client's potential for self-harm, level of coping skills, degree of hopelessness, and use of support systems.

C. Outcome Identification
Outcomes focus on the client's safety, development of positive coping skills and self-esteem, ability to interact with staff and disclose feelings regarding suicidal intent or plan, and the client's willingness to take steps to resolve any relationship or lifestyle issues that increase the risk of suicide.

D. Planning and Implementing Interventions
1. Suicide Prevention
Nursing interventions focus on the prevention of self-destruction and are classified as primary, secondary, and tertiary prevention depending on risk factors identified during assessment.
2. Suicide Precautions
Clients at risk for suicide need either constant (one-to-one visual supervision) or close observation (visual checks every 15 minutes) in a safe, secure environment.
3. No-Suicide Contracts
Contracting with the client to try and agree to control suicide impulses or to contact a nurse before attempting suicide must be used with caution. Contracts are often made with clients whose suicidal risks are underestimated.
4. Seclusion and Restraint
The use of restraints and seclusion is considered to be an intervention of last resort. Because they can be dangerous interventions and require one-to-one monitoring, they must be used with caution for individuals who are suicidal.
5. Medication Management
Use of psychotropic medications to manage behavior is referred to as chemical restraint. Injections may be required. The nurse must monitor the client's response to medication, including any adverse side effects.
6. Assistance Meeting Basic Human Needs
Clients at risk for suicide often neglect personal care. The nurse provides assistance with ADL until the client is able to be responsible for self.
7. Interactive Therapies
A variety of interactive therapies are helpful to assist the client in exploring reasons behind suicidal ideation and to provide stabilizing support.
8. Continuum of Care
Appointments are scheduled to continue with interactive therapies and medication management as needed. Support services, such as a 24-hour suicide hotline, are discussed with the client.

E. Evaluation
Evaluation of the client's progress in attaining expected outcomes is an ongoing process; the client's mood, affect, and behavior may

fluctuate quickly and unpredictably. Reassessment includes reevaluation of the goals of therapy, the effectiveness of interventions, and the progress the client is making.

V. SUICIDAL ADOLESCENTS
The emergency room is a pivotal point in working with suicidal adolescents. Importance is placed on risk assessment, calling the child or adolescent after a missed appointment, family therapy, and working with teen's school counselors.

VI. PSYCHOLOGICAL AUTOPSY
Psychological autopsy is an interaction with staff to review the client's behaviors and suicidal act. It is used to examine what clues, if any, were missed so staff members can learn from the evaluation of a particular situation.

VII. POSTVENTION FOR BEREAVED SURVIVORS
Survivors of a successful suicide attempt are also victims. Postvention is a therapeutic program for bereaved survivors of a suicide. Emphasis is placed on one unusual dynamic associated with suicide—that is, often the nonfamily members may be more closely involved in the death than the spouse, children, siblings, or parents of the victim. Postvention provides immediate contact with the survivors (within 24 hours) for assistance in coping with their feelings of shock and grief. During postvention with child survivors, the following are helpful: allow the child to express feelings; assist the child to develop meaningful relationships with others; teach the child assertiveness; allow the child to develop ideas and values.

VIII. EUTHANASIA/PHYSICIAN-ASSISTED SUICIDE (PAS)
The nurse is ethically bound to protect clients who are at risk for self-harm. Many clients who are at high risk, however, may request assistance in the consideration and implementation of their wish to die. Care of severely ill clients is derived from explicit, clinically, and ethically sound principles of medicine and not based on uncertain motives, incorrect information, or prejudicial attitudes.

KEY WORDS

Alexithymia
Euthanasia
Lethality
No-suicide contract

Physician-assisted suicide
Postvention
Psychological autopsy
Self-destructive behavior

■ Classroom Teaching Strategies

1. Have students brainstorm during class, and write on the blackboard every term and idea you can think about that has to do with suicide in our country. What have you heard about suicide? How is suicide viewed in America? In your state and local area? Are there things you have been taught or heard or understand about suicide? Use the blackboard terms and ideas to stimulate discussion about the way suicide is viewed in America and in the students' local geographic area.

2. Ask students to seek information on the Internet, in the media, and any other source about suicide in cultures other than mainstream American culture (i.e. Indian, Middle-Eastern, African American, etc.). Compare and contrast these multicultural attitudes and values to those of your students.

3. Present the following scenario to students: "You have been assigned to work with Jamie, a 19-year-old male who has been admitted to your acute inpatient psychiatric unit. Last night, Jamie was admitted at 1:25 AM after being brought in by ambulance from home. He had attempted to hang himself with a rope in the basement of his parents' house. Jamie appears disheveled, smells of body odor, and has a very deep red mark around his neck. When you ask Jamie to sit down and talk with you, he scowls at you and says, "What now?." Develop the following for presentation to your classmates: 1) a comprehensive nursing assessment of Jamie; 2) nursing diagnoses for the first 24 hours of care; and 3) a 24-hour care plan that includes interventions and their evaluation.

4. Susan Smith is a 25-year-old school teacher who successfully completed suicide 2 days ago by shotgun. She is survived by her husband, Brad, and two children, Jenny (age 5) and Steven (age 15 months). Have students prepare a plan of care for the immediate family (the husband and two children). Discuss needs and feelings of suicide survivors within the first few days after the suicide. Use class discussion to illustrate and emphasize the fact that survivors need immediate postvention and support, as well as longer-term follow-up. Discuss the nursing role in assisting survivors of suicide to cope with the trauma of losing their loved one in this way. Also, discuss the importance of providing developmentally appropriate postvention for family members, depending on their age and developmental level.

5. Have students consider their own personal thoughts and philosophy of suicide and self-destructive behaviors. Have them jot down on paper any terms that come to mind. Ask for volunteers to share some of their thoughts and feelings. Use the class discussion to provide students with an opportunity to talk about how they view suicide and self-destructive behaviors. Gently challenge myths and misunderstandings they may have, and encourage the class to reflect upon and discuss these issues.

CHAPTER 29

Clients With a Dual Diagnosis

■ Chapter Summary

The term *dual diagnosis* is used to designate mentally ill clients who show a comorbid chemical dependency or abuse. Several acronyms are used to describe dual diagnosis: MICAA (mentally ill chemically abusing and addicted); MICA (mentally ill and chemically affected); and CAMI (chemical abusing and mentally ill). Five categories have been developed to describe the dually diagnosed client. These categories enable clinicians to assess and intervene with clients, using interventions that are appropriate to their specific symptoms and clinical picture. The nursing process is reviewed, including nursing assessment, nursing diagnosis, outcome identification, planning and interventions, and evaluation. Phases of treatment for this population include: acute stabilization; engagement; prolonged stabilization; rehabilitation and recovery; and the long-term continuum of care. Providing care to the dually diagnosed client is often complex and challenging.

■ Chapter Outline

I. CAUSES
One theory related to the development of a dual diagnosis is the "vulnerability model," based on the assumption that drug use causes a mental disorder. The second model, "self-medication hypothesis," is based on the assumption that individuals with a psychiatric disorder use drugs to help them feel calmer or to counter various clinical symptoms.

II. CLIENT CHARACTERISTICS
Clients with dual diagnosis are characterized as being dissatisfied with life experiences, having inadequate or ineffective support systems, living in a nontherapeutic home environment, and having a history of self-medication.

III. CLASSIFICATION OF DUALLY DIAGNOSED CLIENTS
Five categories have been defined to describe the dually diagnosed client:

1. Category 1: Primary diagnosis is mental illness.
2. Category 2: Primary diagnosis is substance abuse.
3. Category 3: Mental illness and substance abuse occur simultaneously.
4. Category 4: Substance abuse precipitates the onset of a primary mental disorder.
5. Category 5: Substance abuse occurs as a result of self-medication by a mentally ill client.

IV. THE NURSING PROCESS
   A. Assessment
      Clients with dual diagnoses are difficult to assess because they are not a homogenous group and often are poor historians. The nurse must delineate the relative contribution of each diagnosis to the severity of the current symptoms presented and prioritize data accordingly.
   B. Nursing Diagnoses
      Differences in philosophies and approaches of treatment models for mental illness and chemical dependency can affect the formulation of nursing diagnoses, statements of outcome, planning interventions, and evaluation.
   C. Outcome Identification
      Outcomes focus on the client's willingness to participate in treatment, including compliance with the plan of care.
   D. Planning and Implementing Interventions
      Treatment is available in a variety of settings, including inpatient psychiatric units, inpatient chemical dependency units, community mental health centers, and day and evening programs. Phases of treatment are as follows:
      1. Acute Stabilization
         Provision of a safe environment for clients who are at risk for suicide or homicide, are psychotic, or have clinical symptoms of other serious psychiatric disorders.
      2. Engagement
         Involves establishing a treatment relationship, educating the client, providing interventions to enable the client to maintain stabilization, and preventing relapse.
      3. Prolonged Stabilization
         Engagement interventions continue; client discusses potential crises and explores crisis management skills.
      4. Rehabilitation and Recovery
         Client is encouraged to return to work or is referred to community vocational rehabilitation. Participating in self-help groups and establishing a positive support network are encouraged.

5. Continuum of Care
   Begins during rehabilitation and recovery and continues throughout treatment.

E. Evaluation
   Evaluation can be challenging due to the potential for relapse or recidivism. Evaluation focuses on compliance by the client, the stated outcomes, effectiveness of interventions, and progress the client is making.

KEY WORDS

CAMI

Dual diagnosis

MICA

MICAA

Self-medication hypothesis

Vulnerability model

■ Classroom Teaching Strategies

1. Divide the class in half. Assign half the class to develop and present a brief example and definition of a client who is classified as MICAA or MICA. Have them include symptoms and diagnoses. Assign the other half to do the same for a client who is classified as CAMI. Use the presentations to compare and contrast the two approaches to these clients, and the differences and similarities in their symptomatology and treatment.

2. Elicit discussion by the class about societal views of dual diagnosis. Discuss stereotyping, common attitudes, and reasons why these clients may not be able to receive the medical and psychiatric treatment that they need. Encourage students to try and imagine what life would be like trying to live with a dual diagnosis. Include a discussion about the impact of dual diagnosis on the family.

3. Stage a debate in class, with one half of the class arguing that dual diagnoses are a result of the vulnerability model and the other half arguing that they are a result of self-medication efforts of clients. Use the debate to highlight attitudes and opinions about these two theoretical views, and how these attitudes might affect the provision of health care to this population.

4. Ask students to prepare brief clinical examples of clients who may be classified according to the five categories (category 1: primary diagnosis is mental illness; category 2: primary diagnosis is substance abuse; category 3: mental illness and substance abuse occur simultaneously; category 4: substance abuse precipitates the onset of a primary mental disorder; and category 5: substance abuse occurs as a result of self-medication by a mentally ill client). Discuss how treatment approaches may differ based on category.

5. Have students prepare a care plan for a client with dual diagnosis, including nursing assessment, diagnosis, outcome identification, planning and intervention, and evaluation. Discuss difficulties inherent in the nursing care of this population. Discuss the long-term rehabilitation goals for these clients.

CHAPTER 30

Survivors of Abuse and Violence

■ Chapter Summary

Much has been written about the physical and sexual abuse of children, women, and the elderly. Youth and workplace violence has also been recognized as serious and widespread. Child abuse, including physical or sexual abuse and neglect, has become increasingly frequent in the United States. Women are also at risk for various forms of abuse, including domestic violence, sexual abuse, and rape. Abuse of the elderly was ignored, overlooked, or perhaps thought to be nonexistent until health care professionals began to appreciate the extent of the problem in the early 1980s. Youth violence in America is unlike that in any other developed country. Workplace violence is endemic, with about 15 people being murdered each week at work. This chapter discusses the application of the nursing process to victims of abuse and violence. General topics include child abuse, abuse of women, elder abuse, youth violence, and workplace violence. Interventions specific to each type of abuse are reviewed.

■ Chapter Outline

I. CHILD ABUSE
Causes of child abuse are complex and can occur at three levels: in the home, in the institutional setting, and in society.
   A. Defining Child Abuse and Neglect
      Factors involved in identifying child abuse and neglect include cultural and ethnic background; attitudes about parenting; and social, environmental, or circumstantial factors. Abuse is defined as an act of commission in which intentional physical, mental, or emotional harm is inflicted on a child by a parent or other person. Discipline is defined as purposeful action to restrain or correct a child's behavior. Neglect is defined as an act of omission in which a parent or other person fails to meet a dependent's basic needs; provide safe living conditions; provide physical or emotional care; or provide supervision.
   B. Causes of Child Abuse and Neglect: Risk Factors
      Three elements create an environment for abuse to occur: an

abuser, an abused person, and a crisis. A crisis is usually the precipitating factor that triggers abuse by the parent, who is unable to cope with numerous or complex stressors, becomes frustrated, and loses control.

C. Other Characteristics of Potentially Abusive or Neglectful Parents
Characteristics of potential abusers include: depression during pregnancy; fear of delivery; lack of support from family; undue concern about unborn child's gender; birth of unwanted child; resentment toward child from a jealous parent; inability to tolerate child's crying; viewing child as being too demanding. These are often present in high-risk families, but their presence does not mean that abuse or neglect will inevitably occur.

D. Types of Child Abuse
1. Physical Abuse
Common indicators: bruises with no skin breakage; burns; lacerations; abrasions; welts; scars; skeletal injuries.
Munchausen syndrome by proxy: parent fabricates illness in child or deliberately causes injury to gain attention. Shaken baby syndrome: adult loses control and violently shakes a child who has been crying incessantly.
2. Neglect
Neglect is an act of omission, including abandonment, lack of supervision, and failure to meet the child's basic needs of shelter, nutrition, hygiene, clothing, and proper medical or dental care.
3. Emotional Maltreatment (Abuse or Neglect)
May consist of verbal assaults or threats that provoke fear; poor communication that may send double messages; and blaming, confusing, or demeaning messages.
4. Sexual Abuse
Not easily identified because physical signs are not usually seen. Child victims are often reluctant to share information. Episodes are classified as acute, subacute, or nonacute. Three terms are used to describe sexual abuse of children: sexual misuse, rape, and incest.

II. DOMESTIC VIOLENCE
Defined as a pattern of coercive behaviors that may include repeated battering and injury, psychological abuse, sexual assault, progressive social isolation, deprivation, and intimidation.

A. Factors Contributing to Domestic Violence
Factors include: individuals with neurologic impairments, agitated depression, antisocial or borderline behaviors, drug and alcohol abuse; lack of nurturing and mothering during childhood; poor socioeconomic conditions; poor communication skills.

B. Domestic Violence by a Spouse or Significant Other
Profile of abused client includes history of being raised in insecure
living conditions, having been abused as a child, and getting
married when a teenager. Domestic violence takes many forms,
including using coercion and threats; using intimidation; using
emotional abuse; using isolation, minimizing, denying, and
blaming; using male privilege; using economic abuse.

C. Dynamics of Domestic Violence
Three phases of domestic abuse: the tension-building phase, the
acute battering phase, and the loving phase.

III. SEXUAL HARASSMENT, ABUSE, AND RAPE
Sexual harassment is any unwelcome sexual advance or conduct on the
job that creates an intimidating or offensive working environment.
Rape is considered a universal crime against women. Three elements
are necessary to define rape legally: use of force, threat, intimidation,
or duress; vaginal, oral, or anal penetration; and nonconsent by the
victim.

A. Motives for Rape or Sexual Assault
No single rape victim profile. Perpetrators are from all walks of life
and ethnic backgrounds. Several patterns of rape or sexual abuse
have been identified: anger rape; power rape; sadistic rape;
impulsive or opportunistic rape.

B. Emotional Reactions to Rape and Sexual Assault
Rape-trauma syndrome: Diagnosis used to describe a victim's
response to rape, including an acute phase of disorganization and a
longer phase of reorganization in the victim's life. Long-term
reactions may take several years to resolve.

IV. ELDER ABUSE
Considered a widespread problem. Most frequent abusers of elderly are
adult children. Causative factors include: severe physical or mental
disabilities; financial dependency; personality conflicts; and frustration
while caring for an elderly person.

V. YOUTH VIOLENCE
Largely unaddressed by our health care system. Lethal violence and
gang-related violence has escalated due to use of firearms. No single
cause accounts for all episodes of violence.

VI. WORKPLACE VIOLENCE
Emerging consensus on types of individuals who may become violent in
workplace: angry customers dissatisfied with treatment; clients with
mental illnesses; domestic batterers who follow spouse to work; women
experiencing severe premenstrual syndrome; disgruntled older male

employees fearing job loss; juvenile delinquents; career criminals. Stalking involves repetitive, unwanted communications or approaches that induce fear in a victim.

VII. TRANSCULTURAL CONSIDERATIONS
Abuse and violence affect individuals of all ethnic and socioeconomic backgrounds and are not easily predicted by demographic features. Family income, ethnicity, region of residence, and type of metropolitan area are associated with risk of victimization of children. Cross-cultural variability in child-rearing beliefs is great, so it is difficult to define universally applicable child-rearing practices.

VIII. THE NURSING PROCESS
  A. Assessment
    1. Assessment of Abused Children
       Abusive parents bringing a child in for care are usually inconsistent in their story and provide stories that are incompatible with the child's injuries. Assessment includes thorough physical and x-ray examination; inspection of genitalia and anus; oral, rectal, or vaginal cultures; HIV testing when appropriate. Play therapy and art therapy can help elicit information.
    2. Assessment of Victims of Physical Abuse or Violence
       Clinical assessment is important to determine if victim is in any physical or life-threatening danger. Determining emotional status of victim is imperative. Medical history is also important.
    3. Assessment of Victims of Sexual Abuse or Rape
       Assessment is done to determine if any physical or life-threatening danger exists. Some behaviors that are common during assessment include: acute anxiety reaction; depression; or suicidal ideation. Complete physical and emotional assessment is important.
  B. Nursing Diagnoses
     Diagnoses address issues of anxiety, powerlessness, fear, pain, impaired communication, ineffective coping, disturbed self-esteem, risk for injury or violence, or clinical symptoms of post-trauma response or rape-trauma syndrome.
  C. Outcome Identification
     Outcomes focus on reducing anxiety; improving communication, coping, and self-esteem; identifying supports; assisting victim to return to precrisis functioning.
  D. Planning and Implementing Interventions
     The most difficult task for the nurse is to establish a trusting relationship with the victim and family.

1. Interventions for Child Abuse
   The nurse must be aware of his or her own thoughts and feelings about the situation and must avoid punitive and judgmental approaches. Treatment is multidisciplinary, focusing on crisis intervention and treating the family unit.
2. Prevention of Child Abuse and Neglect
   The nurse may help by recognizing early stages of abuse; promoting educational courses on parenting; promoting community awareness programs; and participating in continuing education and nursing research. Nurses must know the legal reporting requirements in their state of practice.
3. Interventions for Victims of Physical Abuse and Violence
   Plan of action should include providing a safe environment and referring acute situations to local law enforcement officials. Intervention goals are to provide emergency medical care when necessary, empower the victim, and enable him or her to regain control of his or her own life. Provide crisis counseling to reduce anxiety and provide supportive care. Display nonjudgmental attitude; encourage verbalization of feelings; monitor medications; formulate action plan for recurrence of violence; give victim emergency phone numbers.
4. Interventions for Victims of Sexual Abuse and Rape
   Many communities have sexual assault response teams (SART), which consist of a law enforcement official, a nurse examiner, and a victim advocate. Primary concerns center around immediate care of physical injuries; preventing or alleviating psychological trauma; and referral for gynecologic, medical, or psychological follow-up.
5. Interventions for Victims of Youth or Workplace Violence
   Developing awareness of the problem and establishing a workplace, school, or community violence program can help reduce the incidence and consequences of violent incidents.

E. Evaluation
   Focuses on the client's emotional and physical well-being following crisis intervention; effectiveness of interventions; and client's progress.

KEY WORDS

Child abuse
Child neglect
Child discipline
Child protective services
Domestic violence
Elder abuse

Rape-trauma syndrome
SART
Sexual harassment
Sexual misuse
Shaken baby syndrome
Silent rape syndrome

Emotional maltreatment or neglect
Munchausen syndrome by proxy
Rape

Spousal abuse phases
Stalking
Workplace violence

■ Classroom Teaching Strategies

1. Ask students to discuss the definitions of child abuse, child discipline, and child neglect. Engage the students in a discussion about societal views of each, how views differ based on one's individual philosophy and approach to child-rearing, and how individual approaches shape a parent's behaviors toward children. Encourage discussion about how child-rearing is different in different societies and/or how child-rearing practices have changed in America since the early 1900s.

2. Ask students to search the Internet, media, and literature for examples of stories about rape or sexual abuse. Use these stories to stimulate discussion about the experiences of the victim, psychological and physiologic. Use the discussion to enhance the students' empathy for the victims of these crimes.

3. Invite a speaker from a local crisis center to come to class and give a presentation on rape and the triage of rape victims. Encourage the speaker to talk about services that are available in the immediate area for rape crisis and violence prevention. If possible, engage students in a discussion about rape, risk factors for rape on campus, and services available to students.

4. While teaching this class, be alert to student reactions to the content matter. It is not uncommon for students to have been the victims of some type of violence, whether it is rape or some other form of abuse. Discuss with students the importance of acknowledging their own experiences and feelings, and provide a follow-up phone number or contact person so that if the class does stimulate students' emotions, they will have a resource.

5. Have students find the unique child abuse reporting requirements for the area in which they may be practicing after graduation. They can locate this information on the Internet. Have students bring this information to class and discuss a scenario in which they suspect child abuse in a practice situation. For example, if they were caring for a child who was admitted for a broken arm and in whom they suspected parental abuse, what would the ethical and legal requirements be? Review the procedure and techniques for further investigation of this suspicion, up to and including reporting the incident to the state child abuse authorities.

CHAPTER 31

Clients Coping With Acquired Immunodeficiency Syndrome

■ Chapter Summary

Infection with human immunodeficiency virus (HIV) has stimulated much controversy and many health care issues since its arrival in the early 1980s. There is still neither a cure nor a preventive vaccine against the illness. Diseases associated with HIV-positive status and acquired immunodeficiency syndrome (AIDS) are pandemic, and the virus is believed to have infected more than 47 million people worldwide. This chapter focuses on the emergence of AIDS as a primary source of concern in the health care community. Psychological effects are discussed, including a four-stage process of adjustment and coping with the diagnosis of AIDS: 1) shock, numbness, disbelief; 2) denial; 3) questioning why; 4) resolution and acceptance. Family dynamics and cross-cultural considerations are addressed as well. The nursing process is applied, and techniques for assessment, nursing diagnosis, outcome identification, planning and implementation, and evaluation are discussed. These are covered in relation to the phases of disease progression: early, middle, and late phase. Caring for clients and families with AIDS continues to be challenging. Further education, training, and support are needed to assist clients in working through this devastating disease process.

■ Chapter Outline

I. OVERVIEW OF AIDS
A virus causes AIDS and AIDS-related complex (ARC). This virus attacks the immune system, emerging in the form of 1 of 12 secondary infectious diseases or two types of malignant cancers. The two most common diseases are *Pneumocystis carinii* pneumonia and Kaposi's sarcoma.

II. PSYCHOLOGICAL EFFECTS OF AIDS
AIDS is often described as a tragic and complex phenomenon that provokes shattering emotional and psychological reactions in all who are involved. The most serious psychological problems affect those who actually have the disease. Most people with AIDS are relatively young,

and almost all have minority status in American culture. The four stages of reaction to AIDS are 1) shock, numbness, disbelief; 2) denial; 3) questioning why; and 4) resolution and acceptance. Isolation, abandonment, and depression are common psychological and behavioral responses to AIDS.

III. FAMILY DYNAMICS: REACTIONS TO THE CLIENT WITH AIDS
The family may not have been aware of the individual's sexuality and lifestyle. The diagnosis of AIDS causes severe psychological stress and trauma for families. Families may respond with quiet anger, confusion, and possible rejection of the client with AIDS and his or her entire lifestyle. In the face of family abandonment, clients with AIDS often develop an alternate family that assumes the support and caretaker roles.

IV. TRANSCULTURAL CONSIDERATIONS
Heterosexual intercourse has become the dominant mode of transmission in several regions of the world, including North America. Homophobia and stigmatization often cause emotional isolation, disapproval, prejudice, and judgments of shame and immorality; even violence may occur.

V. THE NURSING PROCESS
  A. Assessment
     Nurses' attitudes play a central role in the assessment phase, which is often difficult to initiate due to the sensitive nature of this topic.
     1. Early-Phase Assessment
        Major focus is on obtaining data to formulate a care plan and empower the client to maintain a sense of control. Assess for clinical symptoms of anxiety or depression and identify the client's coping skills and supports.
     2. Middle-Phase Assessment
        Focus on assessing the client's knowledge of the disease progression process and treatment options, coping skills, self-esteem, body image, and support availability.
     3. Late-Phase Assessment
        Evaluate the client's mental status; clinical symptoms of dementia, delirium, psychosis, anxiety, or personality change may occur.
     4. Assessment as Secondary Prevention
        Use a nonjudgmental approach when obtaining a history of blood transfusions, drug use, unprotected sex, and importance of HIV testing for clients at risk.
  B. Nursing Diagnoses
     Formulate diagnoses with consideration to the setting for care delivery. Diagnosis can be challenging because of the presence of

psychosocial and neurologic factors that change over time through
the different phases.

C. Outcome Identification
Goal is improving or stabilizing the client's emotional and physical
well-being and empowering the client to maintain a sense of control
over his or her life.

D. Planning and Implementing Interventions
Treatment and management of HIV/AIDS has changed dramatically
as the pathogenesis of HIV infection is better understood and there
are more effective therapeutic agents.

1. Early-Phase Planning and Implementation
Nursing interventions are based on the clinical phenomena
exhibited. The nurse encourages the client to express thoughts
and feelings, assists him or her in accepting the diagnosis, and
reassures him or her that professional help is available.

2. Middle-Phase Planning and Implementation
The middle phase may last for years. Clinical phenomena
include weight loss, somatic preoccupation, and an actual
decline in physical condition. An individualized plan of care is
necessary, depending on the client's symptoms and adjustment to
the illness.

3. Late-Phase Planning and Implementation
Death is relatively near; palliative treatment is provided. Life
review process is therapeutic; grief work around death and
dying. Family members and significant others also need support
during this time.

4. Continuum of Care
Most communities have full-service agencies to provide support
and education to individuals and families. Support groups
become a key element in treatment.

E. Evaluation
Traditional evaluation strategies are effective when stated outcomes
are realistic, attainable expectations. Nurse may need to make
adjustments due to disease progression and development of
comorbid mental illness.

KEY WORDS

AIDS	Homophobia
ARC	Kaposi's sarcoma
HIV	*Pneumocystis carinii*

■ Classroom Teaching Strategies

1. Arrange to show the film "Philadelphia" (starring Tom Hanks) or "And the Band Played On," or assign one of the movies as a homework assignment. Ask students to view the movie and discuss the societal attitudes toward homosexuality and the experience of the gay individual in dealing with AIDS. Elicit classroom discussion about common stereotypes, issues, and beliefs about alternative lifestyles, as well as the importance of awareness of one's own values and beliefs in the care of clients whose lifestyles may differ from one's own.

2. Divide the class into three groups, assigning each group to one of the following: 1) early-phase assessment; 2) middle-phase assessment; and 3) late phase assessment. Have each group outline important issues in the assessment of the individual with HIV/AIDS at each phase.

3. Using the same three groups as above, have each group discuss planning and implementation for each stage. Discuss nursing interventions and techniques that may be helpful to the client and family during each of the phases of coping with AIDS.

4. Have students search the Internet and media for examples of stories about HIV/AIDS. They can include statistical information, new treatments, psychological issues, family issues, and other social issues. Use the stories that students bring to class to stimulate discussion about the view of society toward gay clients and alternative lifestyles.

5. Divide the class in half. Have students prepare a debate, one side arguing that being gay is a choice and is not a "natural" or "normal" state of being, and the other side arguing that being gay is a physical, genetic, biologically based phenomenon that cannot be changed by a person's will. Encourage students to prepare their debate using factual information they gather from reliable sources. Use the debate to illustrate the level of disagreement that exists within our society about these two views of sexuality, and to emphasize the importance of student self-awareness when dealing with this issue.

CHAPTER 32

Elderly Clients Coping With the Psychosocial Aspects of Aging

■ Chapter Summary

The public is growing increasingly sophisticated in its knowledge and expectations of geriatric health care. Nursing has also addressed the issue of health care for the elderly. Gains in longevity and active life expectancy have increased the importance of psychiatric care for the elderly population. Many factors influence the process of aging, including primary or intrinsic factors (determined by inherent or hereditary influences) and secondary or extrinsic factors (defects and disabilities). There are several developmental tasks of aging, such as establishing satisfactory living arrangements, establishing comfortable routines, and keeping active and involved. Psychodynamics of aging include such feelings as loneliness, late-life depression, guilt, and anxiety. Social and cultural influences play a major role in the perceptions of the elderly, and those perceptions differ according to societal and cultural norms. This chapter reviews nursing assessment (including physical, social, and psychological assessment) and barriers to the assessment process. Nursing diagnoses, outcome identification, planning and implementation, and evaluation are discussed as critical components of caring for elderly clients in the psychiatric setting.

■ Chapter Outline

I. FACTORS INFLUENCING THE AGING PROCESS
   The multiple processes of decline associated with growing old are separated into primary (intrinsic; determined by inherent or hereditary influences) and secondary (extrinsic; defects and disabilities).
   A. Intrinsic Factors
      Include biologic and physiologic components such as gender, race, intelligence, familial longevity patterns, and genetic diseases. Personality also influences adoption of abusive behaviors (overeating, smoking, alcohol use).
   B. Extrinsic Factors
      To some degree, extrinsic factors are controllable, including employment, economic level, education, health practices, and societal attitudes.

II. MYTHS ABOUT AGING

There are many societal myths about aging, but they are slowly beginning to fade.

III. DEVELOPMENTAL TASKS OF AGING

A. Establishing Satisfactory Living Arrangements
   If this need is not met, loneliness, anxiety, or depression may occur.

B. Adjusting to Retirement Income
   Retirement may be a time of relaxation and leisure or it may be a time of crisis. Adjusting one's standard of living to a reduced income may be stressful.

C. Establishing Comfortable Routines
   Dependent on the person's preretirement activity level and personality. Many persons have difficulty adjusting to new routines during retirement.

D. Maintaining Love, Sex, and Marital Relationships
   Might be difficult, depending on client's function in earlier life. Elderly people can maintain an active sex life into their 80s and 90s.

E. Keeping Active and Involved
   Characteristics of clients who keep active and involved include: desire to leave a legacy; desire to share knowledge and experience with younger generations; increased emotional investment in environment; increased creativity and curiosity; and satisfaction with life.

F. Staying in Touch With Other Family Members
   Many elderly people are lonely because they have no family or supports. Loneliness may lead to depression. It is important to sustain these relationships or develop new ones.

G. Sustaining and Maintaining Physical and Mental Health
   Various emotional and behavioral reactions occur as people undergo the physiologic changes of the aging process. Reactions include anxiety, frustration, fear, depression, loneliness, stubbornness, decreased independence and productivity, and low self-esteem.

H. Finding Meaning in Life
   The elderly often reminisce as they adapt to aging. Ego transcendence is a positive approach to finding meaning in life. Ego preoccupation is resignation to aging, inactivity, feeling that one has no future and wants to die.

IV. PSYCHODYNAMICS OF AGING

Erikson's (1963) last stage of psychological development is identified as ego integrity versus despair. Failure to thrive can occur, in which the client has unexplained weight loss, deterioration in mental status and functional ability, and social isolation.

A. Anxiety
Loss of mental acuity, placement in nursing home, loss of spouse, emergency surgery, diagnosis of illness are causes of anxiety in old age.

B. Loneliness
Elderly often feel lonely due to death of spouse, friends; loss of pet; inability to communicate in English; pain; certain times of day or night.

C. Guilt
Guilt feelings may emerge from past conflicts or regrets.

D. Late-Life Depression
Depression appears to increase in degree and frequency during old age. Medications may also begin or enhance a depressive reaction.

E. Somatic Complaints
Hypochondriasis, or preoccupation with one's physical and emotional health, resulting in bodily or somatic complaints, is common in the elderly.

F. Paranoid Reactions
Aging persons may feel that others are talking about them or conspiring against them. Medications may also precipitate these feelings.

G. Dementia
Dementia is an acquired, organic syndrome defined by the presence of cognitive deficits such as memory impairment and problems with abstract thinking and judgment. The elderly are at risk for dementia and should be assessed frequently. Depression is the most frequent psychiatric disorder associated with dementia in the elderly.

H. Delirium
Characterized by a disturbance of consciousness and impairment of attention that fluctuates during the day. It is particularly important to identify delirium because it is assumed to be a reversible disorder.

V. TRANSCULTURAL CONSIDERATIONS
Culture defines who is "old," establishes rules for identifying the elderly, sets socially acceptable roles and expectations for behavior in the elderly, and influences attitudes toward the aged.

VI. THE NURSING PROCESS
A. Assessment
Assessment of elderly clients is multifaceted, focusing on collection of demographic data, interview process, and review of medical records. Goals in assessment include providing the best treatment and services available to the client, achieving the best possible

outcome, minimizing cost and time, advocating for identified
necessary services, and reducing stress for both the client and his or
her caregivers.

1. Polypharmacy
   Polypharmacy can place clients at risk for a variety of
   physiologic changes, such as electrolyte or metabolic imbalance,
   liver damage, or renal failure.

2. Barriers to Assessment
   a. Provider-Related Barriers
      Concern about stigmatizing the client; uncertainty about
      when to assess for mental health problems; time constraints;
      discomfort with discussing mental health issues with elderly
      clients; lack of provider or referral access; reimbursement
      considerations.
   b. Client-Related Barriers
      Presence of a wide variety of symptoms that are difficult to
      prioritize and diagnose; cultural factors; client's discomfort
      in using words such as sadness or depression; possible
      amplification of somatic symptoms for secondary gain.
   c. Illness-Related Barriers
      Presence of multiple factors such as acute changes in health;
      a heterogeneous clinical presentation; undisclosed drug or
      alcohol use; unmet psychosocial needs.

B. Nursing Diagnoses and Outcome Identification
   Can be challenging because of coexisting medical conditions.
   Generally focus on issues of loss or grief; social isolation; alteration
   in affect or mood; low self-concept; changes in behavior or
   cognition; problems related to eating or sleeping.

C. Planning and Implementing Interventions
   Emphasis is on maximizing the older person's independence;
   preventing illness or disability; promoting, maintaining, and
   restoring health; and maintaining life in dignity and comfort.

   1. Life Review Process
      Useful to help elderly clients address unresolved conflicts or
      reflect on their life purpose.

   2. Reminiscence
      A therapeutic process of consciously seeking and sharing
      memories of past significant experiences and events.

   3. Grief Work
      Loss of a spouse is rated as the most stressful life event across
      all ages and cultural backgrounds. It is difficult to cope and
      work through grief.

   4. Psychodynamic Psychotherapy
      Helps elderly people examine their purpose and goals in life to
      achieve creative and satisfying life experiences.

5. Medication Management
   Medication must be used carefully, with ongoing assessment and monitoring.
6. Continuum of Care
   Assisted living facilities, adult day care, community mental health centers, and senior centers offer multiple interventions for elderly clients.

D. Evaluation
   Nurse determines whether any barriers have interfered with the plan of care. Evaluation includes the client's emotional and psychological status and any changes in care that might be needed. Family is included in this process.

KEY WORDS

Ego preoccupation	Hypochondriasis
Ego transcendence	Life review
Failure to thrive	Polypharmacy
Geropsychiatry	Reminiscence

■ Classroom Teaching Strategies

1. Assign students the task of interviewing an elderly person they know. The interview should include questions about the elderly person's perception of aging, what it is like to become older, and what the elderly person thinks others believe about the roles of the elderly. When students get together in class, have them compare notes and identify commonalities among the answers they found. Elicit class discussion about the themes and perspectives that were identified among all the interviews.

2. Ask students to consider what they will be like when they are 80 years old. Have students jot down terms they believe will describe them at that time. Encourage discussion of students' perceptions of their own aging process and the way in which they may change with age.

3. Have students search the Internet, magazines, and other types of media to find representations of aging. Use the findings to generate a discussion about societal views of aging and how aging is portrayed in the media. Compare these portrayals to how aged individuals are actually treated in America. Discuss how the media may have an influence on the perception of the elderly in our society, and vice versa.

4. Have the class divide into groups and try to conduct a brief session on reminiscence. Instruct students to reminisce about a particular part of their lives and to observe the process that occurs within the group. For example, one group might reminisce about their first day of school, their senior year in high school, or the first year of college. After the groups

have finished, reconvene the entire class. Discuss feelings and emotions that were elicited through the group process, and discuss how this might be therapeutic for elderly individuals.

5. Have the class brainstorm on the blackboard, jotting down any terms or thoughts they can think of that they associate with the words *aging, old,* and *elderly.* Discuss where these ideas and perceptions came from, how they were formed, and the stereotypes that may have been expressed. Use the discussion to increase students' awareness of how the elderly are perceived by younger persons. Also, have students discuss how these ideas and thoughts might have an influence on the way they approach elderly clients and on the way they plan care for these individuals.

CHAPTER 33

Persistently Mentally Ill Clients

■ Chapter Summary

Persistent mental illness is a severe psychotic disorder, persisting over long periods of time and causing disabling symptoms that significantly impair functioning. Several diagnoses comprise the area of persistent mental illness, and symptoms can persist throughout these individuals' lives. Persistently mentally ill persons are often rejected and abandoned by society and their community, even though they are often unable to live independently and frequently need assisted living environments in order to survive. Services in the community and society are scant in terms of caring for homeless individuals, and they often are relegated to jail and corrective institutions. Psychiatric nurses play an important role in the assessment, treatment, and long-term management of persistently mentally ill individuals. The nursing process, including assessment, nursing diagnosis, outcome identification, planning and implementing care, and evaluation, is useful in approaching these clients in a comprehensive manner.

■ Chapter Outline

I. SCOPE OF PERSISTENT MENTAL ILLNESS
About 3.5 million Americans have the severest forms of mental illness, and an estimated 40% of these individuals do not receive treatment on any given day. Persistently mentally ill individuals have poorer physical health than the general population, poor living situations, unhealthy life-style habits, and increased health risks. Delivering comprehensive services to this population is one of the biggest challenges facing the mental health care system. Lack of treatment of these individuals is thought to contribute to the fact that many of them are homeless or in jails.

II. FACTORS RELATED TO THE CURRENT PROBLEMS OF THE PERSISTENTLY MENTALLY ILL
Factors contributing to the current problems of the persistently mentally ill are complex and numerous and include deinstitutionalization and the failure of social services resources to provide for their multiple needs.

III. HOMELESSNESS
Deinstitutionalization as well as the lack of adequate psychiatric and social services and the loss of state hospital beds caused a large portion of the population with persistent mental illness to become homeless. Other factors that contribute to homelessness include the presence of positive symptoms of schizophrenia, concurrent substance abuse, the presence of personality disorders, and a high rate of family disorganization. The crisis of being homeless compounds the problems of mental illness.

A. Special Populations of the Homeless
Today's homeless persons are younger, are often drug-dependent, are in greater poverty, and are more likely to represent minorities. Women who are homeless are more likely to have experienced domestic violence. Elderly homeless individuals are also poorer, are in poorer health, and are more likely to have alcohol use disorders than their younger counterparts.

B. Outreach Services for the Homeless Mentally Ill
Most homeless individuals have had some contact with the mental health care delivery system. Providing outreach services to this population is costly and is often fragmented. Lack of adequate resources for outreach continues to be a major issue in treating clients with persistent mental illness.

IV. IMPACT OF MANAGED CARE ON SERVICES
Managed care has created difficulties in providing psychiatric services to the persistently mentally ill because shorter lengths of stays in acute care facilities and relying on medications as the first and sometimes only treatment is problematic.

V. INCARCERATION
Deinstitutionalization has also resulted in a significant population of clients with persistent mental illness being maintained in jails and prisons. Often, mentally ill individuals are jailed because there are not sufficient resources to maintain them safely in the community.

VI. THE NURSING PROCESS

A. Assessment
Assessment must be comprehensive, including current symptomatic behaviors, self-care abilities, living situation, available supports, compliance with medications, presence of substance abuse, and physical health status.

B. Nursing Diagnoses
The nurse establishes priorities among the possible nursing diagnoses based on the client's potential for harm to self or others,

current symptomatic behaviors, self-care abilities, available supports, and physical health status.

C. Outcome Identification
Outcome criteria are focused on maintaining safety, establishing and maintaining client self-care, establishing client trust, facilitating interaction with staff and peers, and decreasing presence of positive symptoms.

D. Planning Interventions
Interventions are dependent on the nurse's ability to assess the client as well as to establish and maintain a therapeutic relationship.

E. Implementation
Combining neuroleptic medications with a cognitive behavioral and psychosocial rehabilitation approach is helpful in treating clients with persistent mental illness. Psychosocial rehabilitation is appropriate for settings such as the mental health center, partial hospitalization unit, and outpatient clubhouse programs. Basic employment skills training is another part of psychosocial rehabilitation that is appropriate for clients who may desire a job.

　1. Providing a Safe Environment
The nurse establishes a safe environment on the inpatient unit that promotes and protects client safety, including use of suicide precautions, safety rounds, and consistent rules and expectations for client behavior.

　2. Orienting to Reality
Includes techniques such as using a calendar and large poster boards that include unit-based information. Other simple physical activities such as writing or drawing can assist the client in redirecting energy to acceptable activities and can help distract the client.

　3. Promoting Self-Care
The nurse encourages the client to maintain personal hygiene and uses techniques such as positive reinforcement for efforts to improve. A regular routine for self-care helps to structure the client's day and reinforces activities on a daily basis.

　4. Providing Support
The nurse provides support by active listening, and educating the client in order to promote empowerment.

　5. Enhancing Self-Esteem
The nurse communicates respect for the client and identifies areas in which the client has been able to function. Helping the client use problem-solving skills, teaching assertiveness skills, and encouraging participation in support groups are also helpful techniques for enhancing self-esteem.

6. Promoting Physical Health
   The nurse uses a wellness education approach to improve the heath status of these clients.
7. Assisting Family Members
   The nurse uses a psychoeducational approach to provide assistance to families of the chronically mentally ill.
8. Planning Continued Treatment
   Working as a team member is important for the nurse in planning continued client treatment. Coordinating services, such as social services, is also an important component of continued treatment.
9. Providing Assistance for Homeless Clients
   The nurse also uses nontraditional approaches to reach homeless clients with persistent mental illness, including helping to locate housing, improving physical health status, and locating and securing appropriate community supports.
10. Providing Care for Imprisoned Clients
    The nurse working in the prison system assists in case-finding measures to identify the population of inmates with persistent mental illnesses. Important nursing interventions include establishing a trusting and supportive relationship and educating the client about his or her illness and medications that are important for symptom control.

F. Evaluation
   Evaluation focuses on the outcomes of client care and the degree to which specified goals have been met. Recurrence of symptoms is common.

KEY WORDS

Deinstitutionalization

Homelessness

Incarceration

Managed care

Persistent mental illness

■ Classroom Teaching Strategies

1. Have students find out what services are available in their immediate community for homeless individuals. Discuss the lack of services and the types of services that they discovered.

2. Ask students to consider what life would be like if they were homeless. Have them write down ideas that come to mind on a piece of paper, and pass the papers up to the front of the class. Ask a student to come forward and write on the blackboard several of the terms and ideas from student papers. Problem-solve with the class about what the role of the psychiatric nurse would be in helping individuals with these types of

problems. Use the discussion to highlight and emphasize the complexity of dealing with the problems of the persistently mentally ill who are homeless.

3. Present students with a case study such as: "You are working in the emergency department of a large, urban hospital. Mr. T. arrives in the ED, and on assessment you learn that he is 35 years old, has chronic schizophrenia, and has been living two blocks from the hospital under a bridge in a cardboard box for 2 months. Mr. T. is currently not taking any medications and comes to the ED with hallucinations and delusions. He is disheveled, smells of alcohol, and is speaking in nonsensical words." Discuss further assessment that is needed and what the immediate treatment needs for Mr. T. would be. Discuss the nursing role in providing psychiatric care for Mr. T. Use the case study to illustrate the complexities of assessment and intervention with homeless mentally ill individuals.

4. Ask students to discuss the impact of deinstitutionalization on persistently mentally ill individuals in their community. Include the perspective of the mentally ill individual, family members, and the community.

5. Ask students to search the Internet and other media to explore the issue of homelessness in America. What are the issues that they find addressed in these resources? Engage students in a discussion about how they might address the issue of homeless persistently mentally ill individuals. Highlight the complexities of the issue and the impact of homelessness on children, families, and society.

Appendix A

List of Media Sources

- Backroads, 200 Tamal Vista Boulevard, #409, Corte Madera, CA 94925
- Carle Foundation, Carle Medical Communications, 611 W. Park Avenue, Urbana, IL 68101
- Children and Adolescents with Attention Deficit Disorders, 499 Northwest 70th Avenue, Suite 308, Plantation, FL 33317
- Concept Media, P.O. Box 19542, Irvine, CA 92713
- Fanlight Productions, 47 Halifax Street, Boston, MA 02131
- Film Makers Library, Inc., 124 E. 40th Street, Suite 901, New York, NY 10016
- Health EDCO, P.O. Box 21207, Waco, TX 76702-12
- Lippincott Williams & Wilkins, 530 Walnut Street, Philadelphia, PA 19106-3780
- Jonathan Parker's Gateway Institute, P.O. Box 1778, Ojai, CA 93023
- Medi-Slim, P.O. Box 13267, Edwardsville, KS 66113
- Music Designs, 207 East Buffalo Street, Milwaukee, WI 53202
- National Alliance for the Mentally Ill, 2101 Wilson Blvd., Suite 302, Arlington, VA 22201
- National Institute of Mental Health, Public Inquiries Section, Division of Communications and Education, Science Communication Branch, room 15C-05, 5600 Fishers Lane, Rockville, MD 20857
- National Clearinghouse for Alcohol and Drug Information, P.O. Box 2345, Rockville, MD 20852
- National League for Nursing, 350 Hudson Street, New York, NY 10014
- Network Publications, ETR Associates, P.O. Box 1839, Santa Cruz, CA 95161-1830
- Polymorph Films, Inc., 930 Pitner Avenue, Evanston, IL 91826
- Pyramid Film and Video, Box 1048, Santa Monica, CA 90406
- Research Press, Box 3177, Department S., Champaign, IL 91826
- Select Media, Inc., 74 Varick Street, Suite 305, New York, NY 10013
- Mosby-Yearbook, 11830 Westline Industrial Drive, St. Louis, MO 63146
- The Soundworks Inc., P.O. Box 10868, Arlington, VA 22210
- U.S. Department of Health and Human Services, Public Health Service, Washington, DC 21201
- V-C Menninger, Menniger Video Productions, Box 829, Topeka, KS 66601-9908

Selected Websites of Interest to Psychiatric–Mental Health Nursing

Many Internet resources are currently available for those willing to "surf the net." Many public libraries, colleges, and universities provide Internet access for instructors and students. Interestingly, it is not necessary for you to understand the Internet to use it. A computer, modem, and subscription to an Internet provider are necessary. A coach or someone to guide you for a while is also helpful. Most subscription online services provide written instructions and phone support to answer your questions.

Once you access one of the many search engines available through your Internet access provider, you can search for the information you want by typing in a few key words, such as "depression" or "Nursing Process." If you search for "depression" you will access thousands of sites and will be instructed how to narrow your search by adding additional words such as "depression and elderly."

The World Wide Web is a search tool that puts a wealth of information and contacts at your fingertips. Once you access a website you can follow their links to other similar websites that relate to the topic you choose to research. The following is a limited list of websites related to psychiatric reading. Use these to link to new and ever-changing sites.

American Psychiatric Association: http://www.psych.org/
American Psychiatric Nurses' Association: http://www.apna.org/
American Psychological Association Homepage: http://www.apa.org
American Psychological Association Search Engine:
    http://www.psychcrawler.com/
Community Mental Health Systems: http://www.cmhc.com/
Federal Drug Administration: http://www.fda.gov/
Government Printing Office: http://www.access.gpo.gov/
Health and Human Services: http://www.hhs.gov/
Internet Mental Health: http://www.mentalhealth.com
Mental Health Information Source: http://www.mhsource.com/
My WebMD Personal Health Site:
    http://my.webmd.com/index?TO=gen&FROM=Excite&BannerID=text
National Institute of Drug Abuse: http://www.nida.nih.gov/
National Institute of Mental Health: http://www.nimh.nih.gov/
National Institute of Nursing Research: http://www.nih.gov/ninr/
National Institutes of Health: http://www.nih.gov
National Mental Health Association: http://www.nmha.org/
National Mental Health Association Depression Screening On-Line:
    http://www.depression-screening.org/
Psych Central: http://www.coil.com/~grohol

Appendix B

Interpersonal Process Analysis #: _____   Date: _____   Student Name: _____

CLIENT: Verbal and nonverbal communication	NURSE: Perceptions, thoughts, and feelings during the exchange	NURSE: Verbal and nonverbal communication exactly as you remember it.	THERAPEUTIC TECHNIQUE AND RATIONALE: Explain how what you said was therapeutic and why (must reference).	EVALUATION: What you could have said differently to make the exchange more therapeutic for patient (give examples, with quotations).

Example IPA of a Beginning Psychiatric Nursing Student: The First Day of Clinical

NAME: Susan J. Student

CLIENT: B.R.

Date: Unit:

The client and I were sitting in a small room adjacent to her bedroom. It is a private area, where no one could hear our discussion. Just prior to beginning the exchange, I had asked the client if I could speak with her for about 15 minutes. She was somewhat paranoid, and seemed suspicious, but she said that she did not mind if we talked. The unit was quiet at the time, as it was about 15 minutes after breakfast had been served.

CLIENT: Verbal and nonverbal communication	NURSE: Perceptions, thoughts, and feelings during the exchange	NURSE: Verbal and nonverbal communication exactly as you remember it.	THERAPEUTIC TECHNIQUE AND RATIONALE: Explain how what you said was therapeutic and why (must reference).	EVALUATION: What you could have said differently to make the exchange more therapeutic for patient (give examples, with quotations).
"Last night, they came and took my heart out, and I couldn't sleep." (sitting in her rocker, looking up and making eye contact)	I wonder if she is referring to a dream? I feel really nervous, because I have absolutely NO clue how to answer her!!! (I crossed my legs at this point). My palms are starting to sweat …	"Who took your heart out?"	I didn't use a therapeutic technique. I was so anxious I just went with my gut feeling.	I played into her delusion?? Maybe? But I wanted to know more about it. A "who" question seems somewhat confrontative. It might have been better to say something like, "It sounds like that may have been scary." Or "You sound troubled." (reflection). Or I could have also asked about the delusion a little less directly ("How is it that they did that?") (Open-ended question). My nonverbal posture is closed.

"The men who come in at night. They stood over my bed and got into my soul." (when she says this, she looks really sad—her head and eyes go downward).

Now, I'm really nervous. I don't know enough about psych to even be here, much less listening to this ... I hate doing this by myself ... where is the instructor anyway? I wish I could go home. (My arms are crossed)

"Wow."

I can't believe I'm so inept! But what she is saying is so unusual, I am scared ... I'm trying to THINK about what to say, but "wow" just slipped out.

It would have been a good idea to try to go for the feelings about her night, instead of the events (which seem to be delusional). I could have said "How were you feeling?" Another way to go might have been to ask about her soul ... "What is your soul like?" (open-ended) or "Can you tell me about your soul?" or I could have also used validation,

"Let me see if I understand what you are saying ..." I could have used a reflective technique " ... they got into your soul?"

Oops, I just noticed I'm sitting with my arms and legs crossed....
I uncross them, but feel very conscious ... ugh!
I am also noticing that I feel sad when she is telling me this ... I think I might be picking up on her mood???
Or maybe I'm just sad to be here, because it's a sad place and I don't feel comfortable??

"So, you said you couldn't sleep? Are you tired today?"

I tried to go for the "here and now" versus delusional stuff ... So I went for an assessment question about her sleep and fatigue. It seems so much more familiar to me....

I think this was a good way to go (redirecting the patient, and reorienting), so I tried to focus her back on her sleeping and stuff.
I'm going to try to listen for things that I can use to refocus her on the here and now.
I could have also reflected her sadness, which I was feeling, by saying something like, "You sound kind of sad when you tell me this."

continued

CLIENT: Verbal and nonverbal communication	NURSE: Perceptions, thoughts, and feelings during the exchange	NURSE: Verbal and nonverbal communication exactly as you remember it.	THERAPEUTIC TECHNIQUE AND RATIONALE: Explain how what you said was therapeutic and why (must reference).	EVALUATION: What you could have said differently to make the exchange more therapeutic for patient (give examples, with quotations).
"Yes, I am so tired. I want to go in my room and sleep right now." (she closes her eyes)	She looks really tired, is slumped in her chair, her shoulders are beginning to the right. I am beginning to feel less anxious. But, as I feel less anxious, I get the feeling she is shutting me out by closing her eyes.	"You know, you do look tired today. I notice you are leaning over a bit."	Thought I could stay on the topic of my assessment and I'm trying to reflect my observations to her.	I think I'm on a good track with her. I feel much more comfortable with this topic instead of the delusions. I used reflection and observation as techniques. I feel like my anxiety is decreasing and I am feeling more comfortable. I am beginning to think I can handle this. Maybe I could try saying "I see" or "Tell me more"
"Well, I'm leaning over because they took my heart out on this side (pointing to her left breast) and now they left a big hole here!" (she looks very sad and her eyes are closed)	Uh Oh!!! Here she goes again ... just as I am starting to feel more comfortable, the delusional materials come again. I actually felt like we were connecting in reality and maybe we could have a conversation.... Although I notice that she has her eyes closed ... that makes me feel somewhat distanced from her.	"Oh. Wow."	Oh, my Lord!!! I still don't know what to say to these delusions. I notice that when I am really nervous, I say "WOW" a lot ... I need to think of something more professional to say when I am at a total and complete loss for words.	Except "Tell me more" will encourage talking and what I need at these times is a little space to think. I am beginning to think that maybe when she starts to feel we are connecting (and I am less anxious), in a reality-based way, she goes back into her delusions because she is more comfortable ... Maybe she even senses that I don't know what to do and that gives her some space when she is nervous? Maybe closing her eyes is also a way to give herself some space ...

"You mentioned you wanted to go in your room now. What do you do when you get sleepy during the day?"	I purposefully ignored the delusional content and brought it back to reality. I think this was a very good maneuver.	Although what I said was good, I could have also gone for the feeling I am getting from her. I could have said, "When you say that, you look very sad. Are you feeling sad?" or maybe I could have said "It sounds as if your heart is sad ..." or "It sounds like your chest feels empty and sad?" All of these things would have been a way to empathize, validate, and reflect, which I'm trying to do to connect with her because it's my first time meeting her.

The discussion ended shortly after the last entry above. I told B.R. that I appreciated her spending time with me. I asked her how it had been talking with me, to which she replied "OK." I made an arrangement to stop to check in on her in about half an hour.

Instructor's Resource Manual to Accompany
Shives' Basic Concepts of Psychiatric–Mental Health Nursing, fifth edition

Installation Instructions

Insert the CD into the CD-ROM drive on your PC.

There are several ways to view the contents of the CD:
- Open the Start menu, go to Programs, then go to Windows Explorer. Windows Explorer will open, and you will see the icon for the CD-ROM drive on the left side of the screen. Click on the icon and the contents of the CD will appear on the right side of the screen.
- On your desktop, double-click on the "My Computer" icon. Then double-click on the icon for the CD-ROM drive. A new window will pop up with the contents of the CD.
- Hold down the Window key on your keyboard and tap the "E" key. Windows Explorer will open, and the icon for the CD-ROM drive will be on the left side of the screen. Click on the icon and the contents of the CD will appear on the right side of the screen.

Double-click on any folder to view the files inside the folder.

Double-click on any file to view its content.

In order to view some of the files on this CD, Adobe Acrobat Reader* must be installed on your PC. It is included on this CD. You will need a word-processing program (eg, MS Word or Word Perfect) to open other files on the CD.

If you currently do not have Acrobat Reader installed on your PC
- Double-click on the folder entitled "Adobe Acrobat Reader."
- Double-click on **ar500enu.exe** to launch the program. Follow the instructions on the screen to complete the installation.

*Copyright 2001. Adobe Acrobat Reader is a product of Adobe Systems, Inc. All rights reserved.